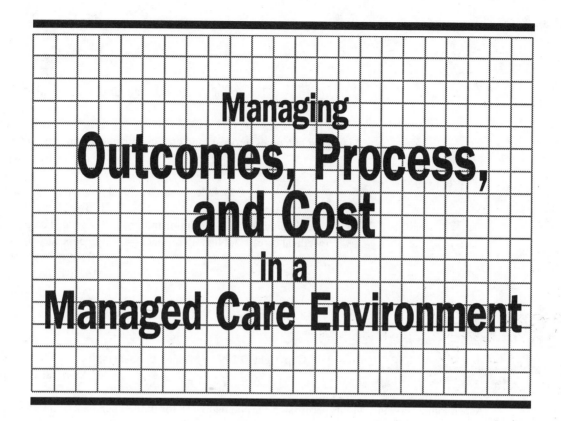

Managing
Outcomes, Process, and Cost
in a
Managed Care Environment

Roey Kirk, MSM, CHE
President ♦ Roey Kirk Associates
Miami, Florida

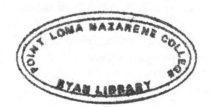

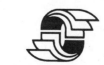

AN ASPEN PUBLICATION®
Aspen Publishers, Inc.
Gaithersburg, Maryland
1997

Library of Congress Cataloging-in-Publication Data

Kirk, Roey.
Managing outcomes, process, and cost in a managed care environment
Roey Kirk.
p.   cm.
Includes bibliographical references and index.
ISBN 0-8342-0912-8
1. Nursing services—Administration.   2. Managed care plans
(Medical care)   3. Nursing services—Quality control.   I. Title.
RT89-K559   1997
362.1'73'068—dc21
96-48673
CIP

Aspen Publishers, Inc., grants permission for photocopying for limited personal or internal use.
This consent does not extend to other kinds of copying, such as copying for general distribution,
for advertising or promotional purposes, for creating new collective works, or for resale.
For information, address Aspen Publishers, Inc., Permissions Department,
200 Orchard Ridge Drive, Suite 200, Gaithersburg, Maryland 20878.

Orders: (800) 638-8437
Customer Service: (800) 234-1660

About Aspen Publishers • For more than 35 years, Aspen has been a leading professional publisher in a variety of
disciplines. Aspen's vast information resources are available in both print and electronic formats. We are committed
to providing the highest quality information available in the most appropriate format for our customers. Visit Aspen's
Internet site for more information resources, directories, articles, and a searchable version of Aspen's full catalog,
including the most recent publications: **http://www.aspenpub.com**
Aspen Publishers, Inc. • The hallmark of quality in publishing
Member of the worldwide Wolters Kluwer group

Editorial Resources: Marsha Davies
Library of Congress Catalog Card Number: 96-48673
ISBN: 0-8342-0912-8

Printed in the United States of America

1   2   3   4   5

for blair juli jones
a challenging distraction... a joyful inspiration... a cherished treasure

Table of Contents

Life is either a daring adventure... or nothing. – Helen Keller

Sometimes, nothing looks *very* attractive. So many challenges, so many learning opportunities, so many nights spent at the office... managers are the shock absorbers of the healthcare industry. Patients, families, businesses, payers, and physicians want the best of the best available care. At the same time, these same customers are clamoring, demanding lower costs. Who's responsible? Management. This book is about what managers can do.

One's first instinct is to go back to the bedside, to stop planning, organizing, leading, staffing, and evaluating, and start doing. In the short term, it's fine, but in the long term the care and service outcomes will be compromised. We need our managers to manage. Planning and leading will reliably lead to better results. Organizing and staffing for a particular workload through process and system design provide staff members with guidelines on how to achieve outcomes efficiently and effectively. Creating indicators as measures and assessing performance results provide management with useful evaluation information to use for decision making and problem solving.

Many of us in the healthcare industry came into management positions using the "POOF" method. We were great technical caregivers or service providers and one day a senior manager bopped us on the head with a magic wand and said "Poof, you're a manager." Most of us did not go to courses or school to learn to be a manager and those of us who did were often frustrated with the amount of practical application offered.

As the leadership of the organization—as well as subject matter experts—managers can multiply whatever they have to offer at the bedside or point of service, using the methods, skills, and guides offered in this book. The applications are intentionally easy. They have been tested by hundreds of users. They are efficient and facilitate efficiency in any team. In a nutshell, they help managers get the job done through and with other people. The material was designed to allow the reader to jump in at any point or to read in sequence.

My goal was to simplify a variety of management skills and methods in order to give managers a repertoire of options that will be helpful in very challenging times ahead. The fact that you are reading this preface, is why I do it, and why I know we'll be successful. Although healthcare managers may occasionally pout, whine, and complain, I know of no other group who care so much or work so hard. And while there is a lot on our plates at the moment, there is also a lot at stake, and there are many opportunities. I hope this book will help you turn your knowledge, enthusiasm, and frustration into positive action and results. Enjoy the adventure.

There is only one name on this book, but there's an army who made it happen. You know who you are... students, workshop participants, clients, colleagues, and brain-pickers who phoned for "reality checks." Because of you, I've been able to write a customer driven and focused book. Every question, every attempt to help me understand how your situation was different, every frustration you described has helped this book become a reality. You all have pushed me to grow, to learn, to research, and to examine my own assumptions and beliefs... and for this, I thank you. I could not have done it without you.

Some were extraordinarily generous...

Helen Hoesing - You gave me time you did not have, energy that should have been spent on yourself, access to your vast knowledge and experience, and wisdom that elevated this book to a whole new level.

Susan Todaro Tumarkin - You gave me time you did not have, an extraordinarily quick turnaround of work I did not deserve, and meaningful information that bridged the gap between payer and provider.

Lyle Greenfield - Thanks for the emergency writing assistance.

All of you who contributed to the "First Annual Be-in-Roey's-Last-Book Contest," helped by bringing your own reality and experience to the examples, an invaluable gift for readers who are walking in your shoes. You also gave me time you did not have (note the trend). You are all mentioned by name next to your individual contributions.

I'd also like to thank my personal support team:

To my husband, Jeff Jones - Thank you for your support and love, for proofreading, critiquing art, listening, and encouraging. You always come through for me and always exceed my expectations. I treasure you.

To my dad, Buddy Blair - Thank you for your unwavering enthusiasm and belief in me and my ability. Throughout my life, you modeled and taught me the value of doing the right things right. As they say in the biz, you walked the talk.

To my friend, Lyanette Gaulion - More than you could know, you saved this book. Thanks for hanging out with Blair, keeping her busy—and happy—so I could work with less guilt. Thanks, too, for the times you chose photocopying over rollerblading.

PLAN:

A PICTURE OF
A FUTURE VISION,
PAINTED BY A TEAM

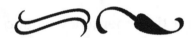

PLANNING:

THE PIVOTAL STEP
IN THE PROCESS OF
GETTING THERE

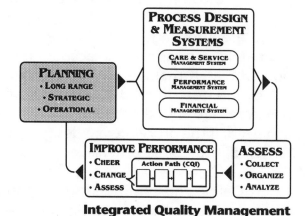

Integrated Quality Management

1. PLANNING

Introduction

If you're a healthcare manager, you
know the rub—you're trying to manage within the constraints of reimbursement ceilings, budget cuts, and too little staff—and you can't help wondering at what point clinical and service outcomes will be sacrificed for the sake of productivity and profitability targets. Your concerns are valid. If you're budgeted for 1.5 hours of care per average **modality** (e.g., test, procedure, visit), and, somehow, a lot of high-acuity and time-consuming modalities all end up scheduled for the same day, you might really need 2.0 care hours per modality (HPM). Staff members might find themselves trying to squeeze 10 hours of care into an 8-hour day or taking shortcuts on care.

As a manager, you are responsible for avoiding either of these inappropriate responses. Both cross-functional and department-specific (natural) work teams need other, more acceptable alternatives, as well as more control over how they use their time. Most important, they need reliable *methods* to help them determine and structure a realistic, achievable workload in advance. It is easy to say "Redesign your workflow and eliminate steps," or "Ensure high-quality care within cost constraints." However, the task of accomplishing these goals while maintaining employee satisfaction is a painstaking and delicate challenge. The most successful solutions have come from those who participate in the process on a day-to-day basis—the real subject matter experts: managers and their employees.

Outcomes, Process, Cost

In an uncertain healthcare industry, there are two things we know as fact. One, regardless of the decision maker (government, managed care companies, individuals, or businesses), cost constraints will continue to tighten. Two, as data become more available and more reliable, they will increasingly be used in decisions relating to quality. Data will drive *how* we deliver care. Data will drive improvement opportunities. Data will drive competition strategies. Healthcare organizations that can show data verifying they provide the best quality outcomes at the lowest cost will be in the best position to compete for their share of the market.

If you are a manager, it all begins—and ends—with you. Management is ultimately responsible, and accountable, for quality *outcomes*. In collaboration with staff members, management is responsible for developing processes and systems for delivering care and related services to patients. If the processes are sound and employees follow them, targeted results will be achieved. If the processes are designed to use resources most efficiently, the targeted results will be achieved at the lowest possible cost.

1. Define and communicate outcomes.
2. Assess and design (or redesign) processes.
3. Effectively and efficiently use resources.

It's a three-stage process that sounds easy and reasonable, but there is a lot of work behind the words—management's work.

Total Quality Management Model

Excellent organizations function well because the leadership of the organization creates a plan for excellence and then carries out the plan. An organization's well-being should never be left to chance: Thus, most organizations have a system or model to follow that gives structure to their management philosophy. If, for example, high-quality care (both service and clinical) at the lowest possible cost is a strategic priority, a framework and a plan will help that outcome to be achieved. Many organizations have embraced (and some have unembraced) a total quality management (TQM) model as a system for managing their organization. While there is debate over which model is best, it seems to matter less which model is used, and more how dedicated the organization is to pursuing the selected model. Also, regardless of which management system is advocated, structure is required to ensure a successful implementation of the model. Figure 1.1, **Total Quality Management Model,** combines concepts from many different models and theories. Initially, Improving Organizational Performance was the only element of this

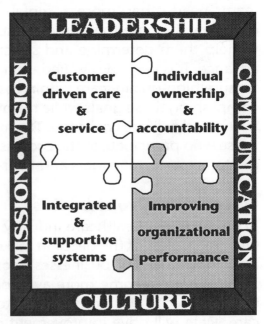

Figure 1.1
Total Quality Management Model

model that was required by the Joint Commission on Accreditation of Healthcare Organizations (Joint Commission). However, current standards reflect the need to address all aspects of this model.

Improving organizational performance (IOP) identifies the need for organizations to have a system in place for *(1) assessing* quality outcomes and their corresponding processes, *(2) improving* quality, and *(3) sustaining* that improvement over time. Regardless of the system of managed care (and who knows what system will be reimbursing in the years to come), providers will need a solid system for improving and sustaining performance levels and documenting them with data. Over the years, organizations discovered that having this system in place not only helped them meet Joint Commission standards, but also provided them with essential business information:

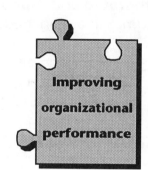

- *How we're performing and why*
- *How our performance compares*
- *Where we want to be*
- *How to get there*
- *If desired results were achieved*

Organizations that know how well they are doing, in terms of cost and quality, clearly have the competitive edge.

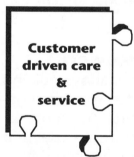

Many organizations pursuing the improvement of organizational performance—including the Joint Commission—discovered that improvement is difficult to achieve without the three other pieces of the puzzle. For one, if you don't know what your customers (i.e., patients, physicians, payers, visitors, etc.) want—or who they are for that matter—it is impossible to pursue performance improvement. Identifying key external, and internal, customers and finding out what they want are two important steps in **customer driven care and service**. Patient-focused care, guest relations, centers of excellence, etc. are all approaches to help organizations find out *who* their customers are, *what* they want, and the *best process* to use to ensure the delivery of excellent clinical care and service.

Likewise, successful organizations know that to achieve the above, everyone in the organization must be part of the process. **Individual ownership and accountability** enhances and multiplies the potential to achieve key organizational outcomes. The accountability loop starts at the top, with leadership owning their own accountability and evaluating their own effectiveness. The creation of high-quality outcomes and a reputation for always delivering on those outcomes require everyone's cooperation. It's everyone's job. Conversely, it only takes one bad experience in the admitting department (or any entry point) to create an angry patient and/or family with accumulating, and escalating, problems for the remainder of the stay. The often-cited example of people walking by a dangerous puddle of water in the hallway, saying, "Not my job," applies here. Patient-care processes involve hundreds of steps and interactions by dozens of individuals. It only takes one action to upset a process and possibly the desired outcome.

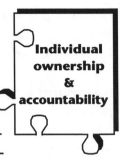

Last, **integrated and supportive systems** are essential to maximizing quality outcomes in a managed care environment. When employees are trying to do the right thing the first time, using the most effective and efficient processes, while organizational systems are not supportive to their task, they may be unsuccessful and become frustrated. For example, one work team was trying to find a way to reduce use of full-time equivalents during low activity periods, but there was a policy restricting, by penalizing, unpaid leave. An organizational *system* was obstructing the team from its goal. Another example: Senior management was trying to promote teamwork within the organization, but all rewards were for individual performance. Again, a large, well-established, organizational *system* was working against the current objective.

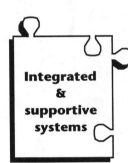

Leadership Responsibilities/Structure (Framework)

Success comes most easily and more consistently when the above guiding principles are supported with an organizational infrastructure. The most essential part of that structure is **leadership** itself. Why? When leadership is involved—deeply involved and committed to—a particular system for achieving high-quality care within cost constraints, targeted outcomes are more likely to be achieved. Also, leadership is ultimately responsible for all four pieces of the puzzle, as well as the other three sides of the infrastructure. For one, leadership plans and formulates the **mission and vision** for the organization (or for the department or function, if the leader is a mid-level manager). Leadership creates the **culture** in which employees can thrive and work toward organizational objectives—a culture that is conducive to risk taking, doing the right things, doing them the right way, improving performance, as well as understanding the value of mistakes

Leadership Priorities

On a personal level, here's what you can do

Create organizational time for learning (all levels & departments):

- Have reading assignments and follow-up discussions • methodical information flow.
- Provide cross-functional chimney-busting • training • contests • involvement invitation.
- Capitalize on uncertainty • take and learn from risks, successes, and mistakes.
- Expand everyone's ability (and accountability) to create and produce desired outcomes.

Clarify expectations of results and process:

- Clarify mission, vision, values • mutual agreement, deployment, and sustained pressure
- State organizational priorities for performance improvement breakthrough • ask, "How can we do things better?"
- Assign process owners for all key organizational processes.

Manage results and process:

- Manage performance and measurement: (1) accountability for cooperative effort, (2) predetermined indicators of success: met, not met, or exceeded.
- Encourage senior team cooperation, customer-supplier connections, agreement.
- Remove obstacles and disincentives, then reward, recognize, offer feedback.

Use hypercommunication: Talk, listen, ask questions, walk-the-talk:

- Know your audience: employees, all customers, the process itself.
- Know key customer forums: employees, patients, physicians, third party.
- Use communication and information networks: TV, computers, bulletin boards.

Protect the organizational environment (we're all in this together):

- Foster good relationships, cultural truths, and trust building.
- Use participative management • task forces • self-destruct or project teams.
- Commit to employees • reconcile individual and organizational needs.
- Share ownership • we're all in this together.

Exhibit 1.1 Leadership Priorities

and ongoing learning. Last, leadership is responsible for **communicating**—through words and action—the mission, vision, and priorities throughout the organization. This is particularly important when policies are implemented or changed because if employees do not see the fit, or understand how policies link to the mission, they may be confused or fail to prioritize their implementation.

Isolated outcomes can, and often are, achieved without top or mid-level management support and leadership. However, it is much faster, easier, and complete when leadership, as a team, is solidly behind these guiding principles, encouraging and facilitating interdisciplinary teamwork. Beginning at the personal level, the list of **Leadership Priorities**, Exhibit 1.1, describes actions that leadership, at all levels, can practice.

At different levels, leadership has different roles and responsibilities for maintaining and maximizing quality in a managed care environment. There are specific actions leaders can take that will create significant levels of success. Starting with **senior management**, the following is a list of actions that will help implement and sustain a quality plan. The list was derived from (1) lessons learned from senior managers who have been kind enough to share, (2) wishes of mid-level managers and employees, and (3) the author's observations of organizations going through this process.

How senior management can help:

- *Effective **communication**: giving necessary information and attentive, nonjudgmental listening*

- *Focused **leadership**: clarifying vision, direction, goals, and priorities*

- *Flinch-free **empowerment**: Backing up decisions and allowing input to decisions*

- *Supportiveness: understanding my department and providing real and visible **involvement** and respect*

- *Pertinent **feedback**: providing information for evaluation and improvement opportunities and recognition for superior work*

- ***Accessible, available, involved**, routine use of **group process** with even, shared participation*

- ***Adequate resources** for the task: providing time, training, space, equipment, preparation*

- Support of a **cooperative behavior** model
- Clearly defined **parameters**
- Effective evaluation of performance improvement system
- Consistent **accountability**: holding managers accountable for performance results

---

Mid-level managers have even more of an impact managing quality than senior managers. When top management is ambivalent, but the mid-level managers and their employees are enthusiastic to pursue superior quality outcomes, some level of success can be achieved, regardless of top management's position. However, a resistant mid-level management can become a tenacious obstacle in the middle of the organization, which, in itself, can lead to severe quality problems. Selling mid-level managers on quality management and performance improvement is rarely a difficult task, however, as they typically want to do the right thing, the right way, the first time and encourage their employees in that direction. Usually, their frustration is with organizational systems that have been obstacles, and they are, thus, often delighted when senior management moves to implement performance improvement plans. Building on the natural enthusiasm of mid-level managers and their staff by setting expectations and clarifying account-abilities will ensure both participation and successful results.

How mid-level managers can help:

- **Use effective communication;** give necessary information, then listen attentively and without judgment.
- **Lead** and **interact** with teams, other functions and departments, and managers.
- Provide flinch-free **empowerment** for employees—earned, appropriate, authentic autonomy.
- Learn and use **group process tools, skills,** and **technologies** to facilitate participation and **involvement**.
- **Identify team leader,** team structure, team members (or selection criteria), and **parameters**.
- Identify the **outcome** and available **resources**, but let team (natural work team or process improvement team) define the process and figure out how to achieve, or improve, the outcome.

- *Create supportive policies.*
- ***Share*** *planning and implementation **responsibilities.***
- *Give ongoing **feedback, recognition,** reward.*

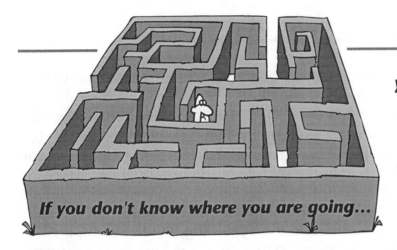

you will probably end up somewhere else.

— *Laurence J. Peter*
Raymond Hull
The Peter Principle

If you don't know where you are going...

Mission, Vision, Values: Planning for Success

MISSION • VISION A second key part of the organizational infrastructure is mission and vision. Laurence Peter's quote, "If you don't know where you are going, you will probably end up somewhere else,"[1] says it best. Unfortunately, most of us have been there and don't want to go back. For those who have pledged allegiance to crisis management and fly-by-the-seat-of-the-pants decisions, or have said, "I don't have time to plan," it's time to acknowledge and accept today's reality that *we don't have time and can't afford to bypass planning.* Being able to do the right things within ever-tightening cost constraints without compromising desired outcomes begins with a clear mission of the organization—its purpose and reason for being—and a vision of what will be in the near future. These and other related terms are defined, with examples, in Exhibit 1.2, **Mission, Vision, Values, Goals, and Strategy.**

Successful organizations use mission, vision, and values to inspire, motivate, and hold members of the organization accountable for achieving the mission. This concept is illustrated in Figure 1.2, **Integrating and Cascading Mission and Vision.** Cascading—or deploying—organizational direction through various levels and functions provides a structure for planning and communication. Planning is always the right thing to do, and the more thoughtful and data-driven the planning is, the better the outcomes will be.

Mission, vision, values, goals, and strategy

Mission: *Broad statement of purpose and reason for being*
What is our mandate? What kind of business are we in, as defined by the organization's by-laws and articles of incorporation? What do our customers need from us? Example: Deliver safe, cost-effective, high-quality healthcare to members of this community.

Vision: *Future image, illusion, outlook, seen on the horizon*
What kind of organization do we aspire to be? What do we want to look like or be in the future?
- *Joint Commission letter of commendation*
- *Market leader*
- *Magnet hospital for physicians and staff members*

Values: *Core ethics, philosophy (often part of the vision)*
What do we believe in? What matters to us? How committed are we? And how will the answers to these questions drive our actions?
- *Customers first*
- *Responsiveness*
- *Cooperation and teamwork*

Priorities/Goals*/Objectives: *Specific outcomes to achieve*
Specifically, what will we accomplish?
- *3.8 out of 4.0 rating on patient feedback surveys*
- *5 hospitalwide cross-functional problems resolved*
- *100% of hospital managers trained in quality awareness and improvement tools and methods*

Strategy: *A plan for accomplishing mission, vision, goals*
Roadmap: How will we get there? What decisions need to be made? What actions? Who's to be involved? Target dates for achievement?
- *Strategic plans*
- *Budget and resource plans*
- *Integrated measurement and accountability plans*

Exhibit 1.2 Mission, Vision, Values, Goals, and Strategy

***Goals**: Many of us have spent time and energy obsessing over the definitions and differences between goals, objectives, outcomes, results, targets, desires, dreams, wishes, etc. If you are one of these people (I'm in recovery) you can stop right here because, to my knowledge—and I've looked and listened carefully for 20+ years—there is no consensus on this issue. I say this knowing mail will pour in from around the world, but it isn't important what you call them, all describe where or what we <u>want</u> to be.

Figure 1.2 also shows, theoretically, the flow of well-organized planning and how it can integrate levels and functions of the organization to help them focus on the same mission and vision. The unity of everyone working toward the same priorities, at the same time, is a powerful force. Even though one group may be performing clinical functions, while another focuses on registration, their unity of vision will help them achieve a common outcome, such as improving outpatient customer satisfaction levels. Notice a change in focus from the traditional cascade—annual goals, divisional goals, departmental goals—to a more direct cascade from annual goals to interdisciplinary team goals (which hold cross-functional teams, as well as the individual functions, responsible and measurably accountable for achieving annual goals).

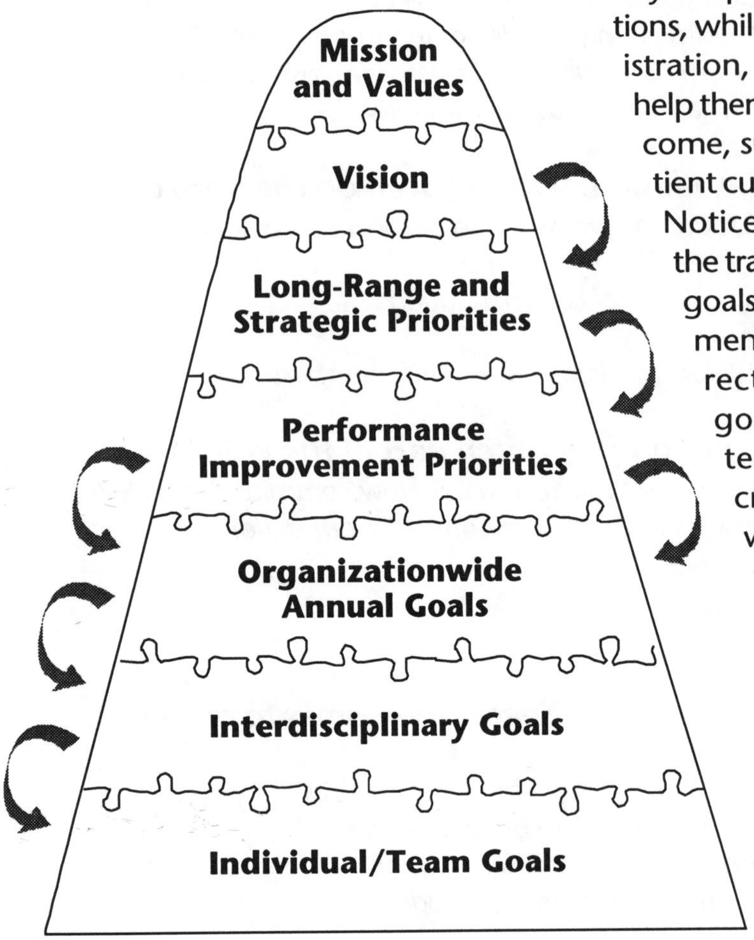

In practice, the concept of deploying mission and vision throughout the organization works in a similar fashion, as shown in Figure 1.3, **Deploying Mission, Vision, and Values** and demonstrated in the example, **Deploying Mission, Vision, and Priorities**, Exhibit 1.3, that follows. The *vision* is translated into a few key organizationwide *strategic priorities* and *performance improvement (PI) priorities*, then annualized. *Annual goals* and contributing *interdisciplinary goals* are pursued, measured, and reviewed by both functional and cross-functional teams so they can *evaluate and predict their potential contribution*. The selected projects may be cross-functional, departmental, task force, individual, or related to a particular clinical pathway, but ultimately all projects link back to the annual and strategic goals that will fulfill the vision and reinforce the mission.

Figure 1.2
Integrating and Cascading Mission and Vision

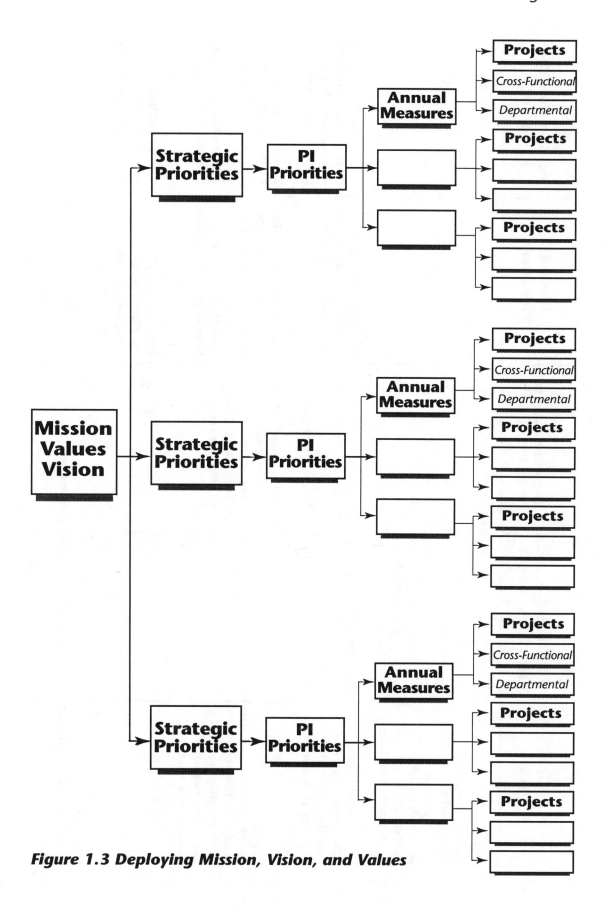

Figure 1.3 Deploying Mission, Vision, and Values

Mission & Vision	Strategic Priorities/Goals	Performance Improvement Priorities/Goals	Annual Measures	Cross-Functional Projects
Mission: To improve and maintain the health of our community through an integrated network of healthcare services.	Strategic Priority #1 Fully functional integrated delivery system			
	Strategic Priority #2 A provider of safe cost-effective care			
To provide accessible, cost-efficient healthcare at the highest standard of quality	**Strategic Priority #3** Improve patient clinical and satisfaction outcomes	**Strategic Priority #3** Patient satisfaction	**Strategic Priority #3** Overall patient satisfaction rating of 4.5	**Strategic Priority #3** Patient Satisfaction Assessment Team Leader: G. Lyanette
		Clinical outcomes	Reduce unscheduled returns to Operating Room (OR) and ICU	Unscheduled return to OR and ICU team Leader: M. Manuel
Vision: To be the recognized leader in providing high-quality healthcare services at a reasonable cost		Patient populations: • Open heart • Myocardial infarction (MI) • Critical care	Enroll all smokers in cessation program	Smoke Enders team Leader: G. Isabel
			Expand use of cardiac rehab program to all cardiac patients	Cardiac rehab expansion team Leader: A. Christian

Exhibit 1.3 Deploying Mission, Vision, and Priorities

Creating the Environment

CULTURE

Most managers are aware that they do not have all the answers (and some have even forgiven themselves). In today's management world, it is not expected that managers have all the answers, but it is expected that they can facilitate "the answers," through problem solving and process improvement analysis with their employees. In an ideal world, individuals are hired who want to do the right thing, the right way, the first time, using the most effective and efficient processes. In fact, this usually happens. However, *behavior,* according to social psychologists, is a function of both the *individual* and the *environment.* Leadership manages both sides of this equation, with responsibility for hiring the right individuals for the available position and creating the environment within which they work.

Although many believe that individuals work best in a competitive situation, there are some very convincing arguments—not to mention some of our own personal experiences—that point to a cooperative environment as the best one for success. Creating and managing a collaborative and cooperative environment is a challenging task whether the manager is a chief executive officer (CEO) or a department head. Fortunately, there are experts in the field to guide us. Alfie Kohn presents a solid case. He notes that in spite of the fact that many of us were raised on notions like competition is good, competition builds character, and competition equals achievement, the reality is that competition can be damaging to organizational results. He believes that when people are forced to compete, they produce less.[2] If you think about it, who can the individuals in our organizations compete against? Only each other, which creates turf issues, internal friction, and lost opportunity to meet customer needs. Another author on this subject, Robert Axelrod, reminds us, "...cooperation can get started by even a small cluster of individuals who are prepared to reciprocate cooperation, even in a world where no one else will cooperate."[3]

If leadership accepts the premise, and responsibility, for creating the environment, then they can choose to create one that promotes cooperation and teamwork. We've all been part of a team (with varying degrees of satisfaction). We have enough experience to know that when there is a sense of esprit de corps—we're all in this together—we want to win, but not at the expense of our colleagues: results are achieved easier, faster, and better. Kohn suggests a cooperative environment could be created by leadership if it focuses on developing the following:

- *Good relationships*
- *Participative management*

- *Shared ownership*
- *Cultural trust building*
- *Commitment to employees*

Reflecting on the above, employee involvement plays a huge role in the cooperative environment, and staff members have a lot to offer, some of which are listed below. However, the appropriateness and timing of the involvement must also be considered and, thus, some guidelines are included for *when to get staff involved.*

——Why get staff—— involved

Staff members contribute:

- *Information, expertise, and clarity about all aspects*

- *Ownership and follow through on solutions and results*

- *Involvement and long-term commitment*

- *Free time for leaders to plan, organize, staff, lead, evaluate*

- *Efficient utilization of resources*

- *Work recognition or reward*

- *Ongoing application of new management skills*

——When to get staff—— involved

Involve staff members when:

- *The decision influences quality, and staff hold the key to achieving quality outcomes*

- *Results can be easily measured*

- *More information is needed, and they can provide it*

- *Their acceptance is vital to results*

- *They support organization goals*

- *The decision could cause conflict*

- *Leaders are secure in their job, their ability, and their knowledge of their staff's capability*

There was a time when involving employees was easier than it is today. For one thing, employees jumped at the chance to participate, to be empowered. For another, freeing employees from their routine work was relatively easy. Last, there was not as much at stake, in terms of results. Usually, if the participation failed or did not occur, it was assumed that the manager was at fault: "Yo-yo empowerment," "Sure, we have participative management around here, as long as you guess the right answer," "The manager would not let go of control," and so forth. Today, there are many reasons being given on both sides as to why participative management or empowerment is not occurring as much as it could be, and because of this, involving and empowering employees in decisions are not as easy as one may think.

The two lists give a good overview of why managers and their employees resist getting involved in participative or empowered exchanges. While management resistance was long thought to be the sole culprit, in today's busy, downsized healthcare organizations, it's more likely to be the staff member who says, "Go away," "I have enough to do," "Isn't that your job?" and "Drop dead."

—Why managers resist...

- *Job or emotional insecurity*

- *Lack of confidence in staff, I can do it faster, better, cheaper*

- *Afraid to make a mistake (unsafe environment)*

- *Unable/unwilling to communicate what needs to be done*

- *Unclear authority (mine/theirs)*

- *Lack of feedback and control*

- *Can't ask staff to do what I wouldn't do*

- *Rewarded for crisis management*

—Why employees resist...

- *Easier, no risk to be taken*

- *Unclear level of authority*

- *Negative environment (no trust, it's just a fad, etc.)*

- *Manager hovering, evaluating, and/or judging*

- *Indecisive employees and/or managers*

- *Not enough information, ability, preparation, or time*

- *No reward or gain*

- *Yo-yo empowerment survivors*

The term *participative management* is not new to most of us. In fact, William Byham, in his book <u>Zapp! The Lightning of Empowerment</u>, poses the question, "Whatever happened to participative management?" He goes on to say, "In the Fifties, managers thought it meant being friendly to employees. In the Sixties, they thought it meant being sensitive to the needs and motivations of people. In the Seventies, managers thought it meant asking employees for help. In the Eighties, it meant having lots of group meetings."[4] Byham goes on to discuss possible reasons for the failure of participative management. However, another, even bigger, issue screams out from the sidelines loud and clear: We've been talking about participative manage-ment forever— fortysome years—and it still isn't established practice! Intel-lectually, we buy it, but emotionally, when there is a shortage of time or a lot at stake, our manager's instinct is to pull in on the reins, take control, and start making decisions.

The fact remains that organizations can do a much better job of improving performance with the input of employees—subject matter experts who per-form and experience processes every single day. Their involvement in per-formance improvement isn't just nice, it's a matter of survival.

Educating, Involving, and Empowering Employees

Empowerment, occasionally referred to as the "E-word," is controversial. It is also a lot easier to talk about than to do. Most managers feel strongly about the subject, however, and this author is no different. Some editorial comments follow:

- *Empowerment is not a yes or no decision*. As shown in Exhibit 1.4, **Empowerment Continuum,** levels of empowerment fall on a con-tinuum that ranges from a completely autocratic decision to a totally empowered decision, where staff members have control over the decision or outcome, as long as it is adheres to preset parameters.

- *Empowerment is not "no management*." In fact, it requires a lot more work and planning on management's part in order to be suc-cessful. The challenge for management is to determine where the individual or group falls on the continuum, so that an appropriate leadership style can be adopted.

- *The amount of empowerment, and, thus, leadership style will vary based on the assigned task*. For example, you may have a group of highly skilled, experienced, and enthusiastic physical thera-pists who are now learning a whole new type of therapy. A manager who previously empowered this group may need to adopt a differ-ent leadership style to help the group be successful until its experi-ence level, attitude, and desire increase to match its general compe-tence. Micromanaging a group of subject matter experts will infuri-ate and demotivate. Giving too much empowerment before an in-dividual or group is ready may leave them floundering or failing. Generally, autonomy is increased as individuals and teams accrue more of the following:

Empowering: a continuum of options

Autocratic: Management decides & acts	Employee input which may/may not be used	Employee input with pre-agreement to use input	Empowered: Employees decide & act

Example #1: One multifaceted situation with varying degrees of empowerment

Decision to purchase a management information system	Suggestions of which systems to study in detail and pilot	Specifications, product evaluation criteria, and preferences	Implementation plan for individual units/departments

Example #2: Same issue (scheduling) with different levels of empowerment

Manager #1 makes up schedule based solely on workload need	Manager #2 schedules, accepts requests, which may or may not be granted	Manager #3 schedules, but will grant all "reasonable" (predefined) requests	Employees self-schedule within parameters set by Manager #4

Exhibit 1.4 Empowerment Continuum

- *Experience*: An individual's or group's actual track record (skills and behaviors) with this or similar work
- *Competence*: General talent, ability, related skills, learning capacity (speed/ease), common sense
- *Esteem/Attitude*: Confidence and belief in self, positive, can-do outlook, willing to risk
- *Desire*: Motivation, interest, or energy needed for new work

• **If not clarified in advance, employees and mid-level managers tend to assume they are totally empowered.** Others think it means a "democratic," or "laissez-faire" decision. Accurate and clear communication is essential here. It is perfectly acceptable to (tactfully) say, "I need your input, which I may or may not use." Then individuals can decide in advance if they want to put forth the effort and won't be surprised, or feel deceived, if it is not used.

• **When given, empowerment should be earned, appropriate, authentic autonomy.** It's all right to select carefully the issues with which you feel comfortable empowering your staff. Some issues will be inappropriate; others, just too close to your heart. Let staff members earn the privilege, then select the issues where they have interest and can make the greatest contribution. Then set parameters, and let them go. Beware: Failing to respond at the promised level of empowerment will lead to frustration, low morale, and refusal to participate in future projects.

- ***Most failures occur because appropriate parameters have not been identified and communicated in advance.*** Parameters are simple limits that help guide empowered teams and individuals. Identifying parameters is, clearly, the most difficult part of empowering a team, but taking the time to set and communicate parameters will save much more time and a lot of disappointment later. At first, it's difficult to anticipate all of the possible obstacles. Thus, the list below might be helpful. Adhering to the parameters minimizes "yo-yo empowerment" and disappointing team results.

Setting Clear Parameters: Some Examples

- *Setting expectations of results, in general*

- *Target cost or cost-benefit ratio*

- *Acceptable amount of time to be spent by the team*

- *Number of team members and, when appropriate and pertinent, who the membership will be*

- *Departments or people to be included or interviewed*

- *Data to be reviewed and analyzed*

- *Resources available to the team (training, labor, supplies, etc.)*

- *Target points to check in and provide feedback to authority*

As stated earlier, managers think they are empowering their employees more than employees think they are being empowered, and employees think they are more empowered than they really are. The self-assessment tool, **Empowering Employees**, Exhibit 1.5, may give you some insight into your own style. Looking at a copy of the assessment that has been completed by one of your staff members may prove fascinating (or painful), as well. It's worth a look. Following the assessment are some ideas on successful empowerment in Exhibit 1.6.

Empowering Employees
Self-Assessment

	NEVER				ALWAYS

Reflecting on myself as a manager:

1. I understand that empowerment is an outcome of leading, supporting, and training my people.	1	2	3	4	5
2. I give people a sense of purpose by showing them how their responsibilities relate to department goals and objectives.	1	2	3	4	5
3. I help employees clarify and define their tasks and responsibilities.	1	2	3	4	5
4. I help people feel a sense of pride and ownership.	1	2	3	4	5
5. I delegate authority for decision making equal to responsibility.	1	2	3	4	5
6. I communicate a person's authority to others.	1	2	3	4	5
7. I establish controls to ensure that the person is exercising his/her authority properly.	1	2	3	4	5
8. I recognize the accomplishments of groups as well as individuals.	1	2	3	4	5
9. I provide recognition appropriate for the achievement.	1	2	3	4	5
10. I encourage and reward risk taking.	1	2	3	4	5
11. I respond negatively to inactivity and indecision.	1	2	3	4	5
12. I give permission to fail, but I stress the importance of reaching standards of excellence.	1	2	3	4	5
13. I ask for feedback from employees on my performance as a manager.	1	2	3	4	5
14. I spend as much time listening to my employees as talking.	1	2	3	4	5

Reflecting on the employees in my department:

15. Employees are competent and can be trusted to perform on their own.	1	2	3	4	5
16. Employees have a positive outlook and are willing to take risks.	1	2	3	4	5
17. Employees routinely ask their customers (patients) for input or opinion.	1	2	3	4	5
18. This department's members function well as a team.	1	2	3	4	5
19. Employees want to be involved in decisions affecting the department.	1	2	3	4	5
20. Employees are confident enough to manage well under pressure.	1	2	3	4	5
21. Each employee knows his/her job and is clear about what is expected of them in terms of performance and results.	1	2	3	4	5

Exhibit 1.5 Empowering Employees Self-Assessment
Contributed by: Kathleen H. Izzo, Trainer and consultant.

Empower Tips

Group Needs

◆ *Involve those who have work process knowledge, skills, and familiarity.*

◆ *Use process and tools for problem solving, continuous improvement, and decision making.*

◆ *Involve those with enthusiasm, commitment, and ownership of the process.*

◆ *Give focused attention, patience, and an open mind.*

◆ *Give or get permission to remove problems and build solutions into processes and systems.*

◆ *Facilitate an end to blaming, judging, jumping to conclusions, and rushing to solutions.*

Communication Needs

◆ *Let participants know the purpose of their involvement (to inform only, influence, delegate, etc.).*

◆ *Tell why the task is important and why they were chosen to resolve it.*

◆ *Give information: Define authority, constraint, obstacles up front.*

◆ *Clarify and prioritize what is to be accomplished.*

◆ *Negotiate expectations, mutually agreeing on realistic results (what).*

◆ *Listen and share ideas, but let teams decide how to get there (process).*

Responsibility

◆ *Accept, define, and share responsibility and authority.*

◆ *Mentor, support, promote, and facilitate increased authentic autonomy.*

◆ *Admit mistakes. Reported errors can be fixed and prevented in the future.*

◆ *Confront resistance. Find out why (it's often legit), and facilitate resolution.*

◆ *Plan controls. Request specific feedback at predetermined checkpoints. React and respond with feedback that is descriptive, timely, and applicable.*

◆ *Negotiate implementation responsibilities with the group and help them make their own individual assignments.*

◆ *Empower, then get out of the way. Don't be an obstacle, and don't forget to DUCK!*

Exhibit 1.6 Tips for Successful Empowering

T/Maker
ClickArt®

Communication: Deal-Maker and Deal-Breaker

At the risk of being melodramatic, the last piece of the Integrated Quality Management Model, com- 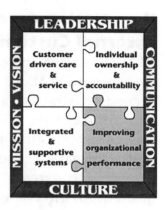 munication, can make or break the achievement of results. Reflecting on the model in its entirety, every element and every part of the framework rely on communication for its successful execution. Still, most organizations acknowledge that communication is a major obstacle to achieving their quality and customer service outcomes.

Reflecting on the Integrated Quality Management Model, and all of its elements, it is easy to see the influence and impact communication can have on an organization. Beginning with the leadership structure, leadership cannot lead, conceive, and share the mission and vision, or create a conducive culture, without communicating effectively with employees. Likewise, the elements of the puzzle, and especially the accountability of the participants, depend heavily on communicating both directions and results.

The importance of effective communication begins with the customer. By definition, customers receive, and suppliers provide, materials, services, or information. Identifying customer needs—so systems can be designed to deliver on those needs—seems simple enough, however, in the healthcare industry, there are many different customers, and this complicates the task. First, there are **external customers**: patients, visitors, physicians, payers, hospices, home care agencies, hospitals, skilled care facilities, and so forth. Typically, but not always, healthcare organizations are pretty savvy when it comes to knowing the needs of the external customers, especially patients. Clinically speaking, it's a necessity. Patients cannot always articulate what they want. For example, in a couple of pages, you'll see some outcome, process, and cost indicators for a laparoscopy. The outcome indicators were created by nursing and ancillary staff, based on their communication with physicians and patients. Physicians provided clinical expertise. The patients' focus was on comfort (were they pain-free and in a private room) and a successful completion of the procedure (did they get what they paid for).

There are also **internal customers**: employees, supervisors, managers, other departments, administration, and so forth. Most employees have not considered each other customers and have behaved accordingly. Senior and mid-level managers are both customers and suppliers to each other at different times. For example, a middle manager in need of a new piece of equipment for his or her department will supply his or her senior manager with the justification of need. The supplied information might be physician request, patient survey feedback, or analysis of the potential return on investment. As the senior manager takes the information, analyzes it, defends it, and budgets for it, he or she transitions from a customer to a supplier of a denial or good news and equipment to the middle manager. Unlike some departments, such as Human Resources (which is usually a supplier) and patients (who are normally in a customer role), managers, their employees, and other departments or functions constantly exchange these roles.

Negotiating Care and Service Outcomes with Internal and External Customers

All of the above and everything we've discussed to this point require effective communication. In order to maximize effectiveness in meeting, and exceeding, strategic and performance improvement priorities, it is essential to work together, successfully, as customers and suppliers. Effective two-way communication between customers and suppliers contributes important information, and while healthcare providers have always been concerned with external customer needs, the internal customer is often neglected. An interview format, **Internal and External Customer Interview** (Exhibit 1.7), has been created to help guide the process. Users have continually been surprised by how much information can be acquired in a very short time. Suppliers interview their customers by asking the written questions. They quickly discover that they are both customers and suppliers to each other and that the interview process can work both ways. The side-bar **case study** demonstrates this theory as well as the intricate interdependence departments (and functions) have on one another.

An Internal Customer Case Study

A lab manager (LM), as supplier, asked an ICU nurse manager (NM) what her department needed and wanted from the lab. She, the customer, said, "We need results reported faster." The lab manager switched into his customer role and said, "Ninety percent of everything you send us is stat. If you could reduce the stats we could turn results around faster." The NM didn't like being in the supplier role because it denoted responsibility; nonetheless she said that her department could reduce the number of stats to 50%, or less, if only the deadline for routine labs wasn't so early. The LM put back on his supplier hat, gnashed his teeth, and asked, "What time would you like?" To which the NM replied 10 AM. Keeping on his supplier hat, the LM agreed and the delays stopped.

Maximizing the customer/supplier relationship is key. Remember, the customers don't care who's at fault when the lab results are late. They only know they're not happy: the physician decision is delayed,

Internal and External Customer Interview

Our service's key customers	**What we think they want from us**
Patient Care Services	Daily delivery of supplies
	24-hour service
Operating Room	Sterilized trays
Emergency Department	24-hour service

Directions:
After you have identified your key customers, arrange a 30–45 minute face-to-face meeting. As the supplier, use the questions below to structure your discussion. Keep in mind that customers often have unrealistic expectations, and you may need to negotiate.

Key customer being interviewed: Patient Care Services

1. What services, materials, or information do you need from our department? You are gathering data for the first column of the *Indicator Development Worksheet*. Probe for specifics (i.e., timeliness, effectiveness [right thing], efficiency [right way], integrity, appropriateness, etc.)?

   Patient Care Services would like the following:
   - routine order and delivery days
   - central supply clerks to stock the shelves
   - to be notified if a product is out of stock
   - to be notified when the product will be available
   - to be told what substitutions are available

2. How does your department use the input (services, materials, or information) our department supplies? This will help me understand your operation and how we can serve you better.

   Patient Care Services uses these materials for:
   - patient procedures
   - general patient care
   - discharge teaching and prep
   - responding to physician orders

3. Are there things we're either (1) not doing or (2) not doing as well as you'd like us to do? We need this information for our department-level performance improvement planning.

   Patient Care Services has been working with central supply to improve our jointly-owned systems, so we're pretty happy. We do fantasize about a 24-hour delivery service for emergency needs and are currently investigating.

Exhibit 1.7 Customer Interview for the Central Supply Department

the patient doesn't get to go home, the patient or the payer has to pay for an additional day in the hospital, and so forth. They only know they didn't get what they wanted, and ultimately, if it happens enough, the organization will pay the price in damaged reputation, unhappy physicians, or loss of managed care contracts.

As demonstrated in the case study, maximizing the customer/supplier relationship requires communication, cooperation, and negotiation. Customers do not always have realistic expectations (as evidenced by the armies of people lusting after a no-calorie chocolate-chip cookie that tastes like the real thing). The more information given to customers, ahead of time, about what can and cannot be accomplished, the more realistic their expectations will be and the more likely the department or function will be able to meet, or exceed, those expectations.

Once internal customers and suppliers have interviewed each other and negotiated expectations, they will be able to prioritize outcomes that each—in their customer role—can count on, and each—in their supplier role—can realistically attain with the help of their staff members.

Indicator Development: Aligning with Customers

Typically thought of as measures, indicators are a great deal more. As stated previously, today's healthcare organizations want to maximize quality and performance results within ever-tightening cost constraints. Individuals want to come to work and do the right thing, the right way, the first time, within cost constraints. This <u>can</u> be achieved, if the following information is known:

- What is the **outcome** (i.e., right thing, target, goal, objective, result, standard of care, specification) to be achieved? What is the direction? <u>What</u> is to be attained?

- Which **process** (i.e., right way, procedure, practice, method, technique, delivery, standard of performance) will reliably, predictably, and efficiently produce the above outcome? <u>How</u> will we get there? What steps will we take? What steps—what work—can be left out without compromising quality outcomes and performance results?

- How much will it **cost**? (1) What is the **avoidable cost**? What does it cost when the outcome isn't achieved and the organization has to pay the price? (2) What is the **necessary cost of quality**? What does it cost, in terms of resource time and dollars, to do the right thing the right way the first time? Unfortunately, in today's market, doing the right thing, the right way may cost more than payers are willing to pay. Organizations must find a way to do the right things the right way within cost constraints.

The **Indicator Development Worksheet**, Exhibits 1.8 through 1.13 is a tool to help managers involve their staff members (the subject matter experts) to integrate outcomes, process, and resource cost and link indicators to day-to-day operations. Remember, indicators are typically thought of as *measures*, but as important, they help teams

- *Design* appropriate work load and the processes to deliver the workload

- *Communicate* information to employees about what they should be working on and the best way to achieve their outcomes

- *Assess* and self-assess performance results and improve

Integrating and Linking Performance Improvement to Operations

A lot of people don't understand, or underestimate the link between performance improvement and day-to-day operations. Some even think the primary value of a performance improvement system is for Joint Commission accreditation. Nothing could be further from the truth. Joint Commission, CEOs, patients, employees, and managed care companies all want the same thing: ***ongoing and sustained improvements in performance (clinical, service, satisfaction) results***. A performance improvement system is simply the organization's designated process for achieving that goal.

Allowing the **Indicator Development Worksheet** form, Exhibit 1.9, to guide actions, the process can be simple and straightforward, as evidenced by the many examples shown on the following pages. They are self-explanatory; however, the **laparoscopy** example highlights several aspects of the tool. It was used by a hospital-based surgicenter to design processes and systems for doing the right things, the right way, the first time. Their challenge was also one of cost constraints. They already knew that, costwise, the freestanding surgicenter could deliver the service at a labor cost of 3.5 HPM, so in order to compete, they would have to keep their costs within that range. Meeting with subject-matter experts (their employees), they carved out specific *outcome* expectations and measurable indicators that would tell them, quantitatively, if they met, exceeded, or did not meet the targeted outcome.

Indicator Development Worksheet

Care or Service Outcome Indicators Care (clinical and satisfaction) or service results	Performance or Process Indicators Recommended process and employee responsibilities	Financial Indicators Necessary or avoidable cost
Human Resources (HR) Standard: Employee education records are accurate and up-to-date. Indicator: 95% of reviewed records will be accurate.	**Student/employee will:** Register with accurate, complete information. **Instructor will:** Turn in all information to clerk. **HR clerk will:** Update computer file information, check for accuracy, backup, and file hard copy for 1 year.	5 minutes 10 minutes 10–14 minutes
Accounts Payable (AP) Standard: All accounts will be paid on time to avoid finance charges. Indicator: 87% of accounts paid by the 20th of the month.	**AP clerks will:** Write checks on the 10th of the month, obtain signature by the 15th of the month, mail by the 17th of the month, and follow up as needed.	1 week out of every month
Central Supply (CS) Standard: Internal customers' needs are met or exceeded by their primary internal supplier. Indicator: 90% of 5.0 scale achieved.	**Internal customers will:** Order on designated days, plan for anticipated needs, and adjust par levels as needed. **CS personnel will:** Restock unit routinely (same day of week/time), note trends in special orders or variance from par level. CS will be open 24 hours for special-needs pick up. **CS staff will:** Assist with unexpected deliveries when possible.	20 minutes 30 minutes Variable
Medical Records Standard: Medical records will be available 24 hours a day. Indicator: 92% of medical records will be returned more than a week after return date.	**Person requesting chart will:** Show identification and sign out, printing all requested info (i.e., phone, return date, etc.). **Medical record clerk will:** Verify information, clarify the return date and penalty, review policy, and offer a reminder call the day before the chart is due back.	10 minutes 10 minutes
Performance Improvement (PI) Standard: All employees will be responsible for improving performance. Indicator: Two cross-functional processes are improved annually, evidenced by key customer outcomes/results.	**Employees:** Actively contribute (team member/leader) to two PI projects (natural work team, task force, cross-functional). **Managers:** Use PI methods to manage natural work team and the team's performance results: use PI tools to manage, interview key customers to identify needs, solve problems, redesign systems, and plan for prevention/improvement.	As assigned 20–40 hours a week Preventing problems and improving performance reduces crisis/fire fighting.

Exhibit 1.8 Assorted Indicator Examples

For each identified outcome, the team analyzed the *process* used to achieve that outcome. Did it work? Were outcomes reliably and predictably achieved? What did it cost to produce this outcome? Was it efficient? After analysis, each process was strengthened to provide identified outcomes at the most efficient *cost*.

After the first rendition, the team came up with 5.8 HPM, which was obviously not competitive. However, since the team was involved in creating both the outcomes and process, they were in a position to reassess their decisions and determine a faster way to achieve the outcome without compromising the quality of their outcomes. This meant eliminating steps. So they went to work, redesigning care (long before there was such a term) until they developed a process that would achieve their desired outcomes within acceptable cost constraints. That sounds easy enough. But it was a real challenge to the staff, who had been providing care the same way for many years without really thinking about *why* they did it that way.

The fact is, over the years, many employees have not had enough control over processes to affect outcomes. Since the process could not be changed, the only control an individual had was staunchly to embrace and adhere to the process, even if it didn't make sense. If organizations are going to be successful at doing the right things (outcomes), the right way (process), the first time, within cost constraints (financial), now is the time to challenge routines, sacred cows, established processes, rituals, and traditions. More will be discussed about this in the next chapter.

Each worksheet that follows represents a body of *teamwork* and *consensus*, not just one person's idea put on paper. Collectively, subject matter experts know better than anyone else (including consultants) the most important outcomes to track, the best processes for reliably and predictably achieving those outcomes on a routine basis, and the costs attached to performing the process.

Indicator Development Worksheet

Care or Service Outcome Indicators Care (clinical and satisfaction) or service results	Performance or Process Indicators Recommended process and employee responsibilities	Financial Indicators Necessary or avoidable cost
### Laparoscopy		
Strategic Priority: *Become the ambulatory surgery provider of choice in the community.*		
Performance Improvement Priority: *Increase volume of ambulatory surgical procedures while maintaining costs.*		
ASSESSMENT • *Baseline physiologic parameters established* • *Ongoing monitoring of changes in parameters*	**Preoperative visit (2–5 days prior to surgery)** • Neuro checks (305.3) • TPR and B/P (305.2) • Breath/bowel sounds (305.4) • History & physical • Preop teaching (301.4) • Blood tests	30 minutes
IVs • *Proper healing without developing an infection from the IV system* • *Administration of fluids*	**Admission, preoperative monitoring** • Preop teaching (301.4) • IV start (444.14) • With piggyback (444.13) • With meds (444.11)	20 minutes
	Intraoperative phase - 1 hour (1 nurse:1 patient)	60 minutes
DRESSINGS • *Prevention of infection* • *Aid wound healings*	**1st stage recovery - 1 hour (1 nurse:1 patient)**	60 minutes
	2nd stage recovery - 1 hour (1 nurse:4 patients)	15 minutes
TEACHING *Patient and/or family are able to verbal-ize knowledge of the patient's care plan during hospital stay and at the time of discharge. This will be supported with a written discharge plan that will include medication prescription and possible complications, when to call physicians, possible setbacks that might occur, etc.*	**3rd stage recovery/Discharge instructions and postop teaching - 1 hour (1 nurse:4 patients)** • Activity goals and limitations (444.10) • Dressing change (331.1) • Medication instructions (432.5) • Nutrition plan (421.3)	15 minutes
		Average total procedure time: 3.3 hours

Exhibit 1.9 Laparoscopy Indicator Example

Care or Service Outcome Indicators	Performance or Process Indicators	Financial Indicators
Care (clinical and satisfaction) or service results	Recommended process and employee responsibilities	Necessary or avoidable cost

Strategic Priority: *Become the cardiovascular care provider of choice in the community.*
Performance Improvement Priority: *Reduce patient readmissions by increasing their knowledge of their disease.*

Care or Service Outcome Indicators	Performance or Process Indicators	Financial Indicators
Knowledge standard: Each patient will receive information related to his or her condition and care of that condition.	**Evaluation standard:** Each nurse will evaluate patient's response and outcomes.	**Resource standard:** Resources will be available and utilized appropriately.
Discharge knowledge indicator: Each patient will be able to verbalize, prior to discharge, knowledge of exercise, pulse, and take-home medications.	**Implementation/evaluation indicator:** Each nurse will document discharge knowledge status in the patient's record upon discharge.	**Resource indicator:** Flexible budget targets met ± 2% for paid direct hours or productivity indicator: 30 minutes (on the average)

Strategic Priority: *Maintain or increase volume of general medical patients.*
Performance Improvement Priority: *Patient satisfaction will increase from 4.0 to 4.5 on a 5.0 scale.*

Care or Service Outcome Indicators	Performance or Process Indicators	Financial Indicators
Satisfaction standard: Patients will be satisfied with nursing and hospital care.	**Assessment standard:** The nurse will assess patient status initially and ongoing.	**Productivity standard:** Care/service will be delivered efficiently.
Attitude indicator: Patient's attitude toward satisfaction is at least 8 on a scale of 1–10.	**Assessment indicator:** The nurse will assess and document patient satisfaction needs each shift.	**Productivity indicator:** 10–15 minutes (on the average)

Indicator Development Worksheet

Exhibit 1.10 Indicator Examples

Indicator Development Worksheet

Care or Service Outcome Indicators	Performance or Process Indicators	Financial Indicators
Care (clinical and satisfaction) or service results	Recommended process and employee responsibilities	Necessary or avoidable cost

Strategic Priority: *Improve and expand pain management and treatment program.*
Performance Improvement Priority: *Improve orientation to pain treatment for patients and their families while decreasing costs.*

Outcome or Desired Goal (patient shares responsibility):	Process (RN responsibilities):	Structure (Time/cost value):
• Attend all scheduled therapies (on time) and update diaries daily.	1. Orient the patient/family to the physical plant.	.5 hours
• Meet with other patients to share experiences and discuss common goals/solutions.	2. Review unit philosophy: self-care, multidisciplinary approach, and importance of group impact.	.5 hours
• Eliminate "complaints of pain" and swapping of medical histories.	3. Help the patient increase control over pain behaviors by providing encouragement, minimizing response to pain behavior, and selective confrontation.	1.0 hours
• Assist other patients to become aware of their verbal and nonverbal pain messages.	4. Support use of learned coping skills (observe & remind).	.75 hours
• Be responsible for using/recording all coping skills used prior to seeking medication. Have a plan to continue at home.	5. Provide audiovisual and teaching aids that support and demonstrate benefits of proper use of coping skills.	.25 hours
• If on detox, report all signs of withdrawal (irritability, diarrhea, nausea, shakiness, headache).	6. Contract with patient to minimize/stop use of narcotics and other nonnarcotic medications, discuss dependency issues, and reinforce use of medication diary.	.5 hours
• State appropriate reasons to contact physician.	7. Discuss the possibility of and plans for coping with a temporary setback after discharge.	.5 hours
• Be able to state side effects of medication.	8. Review attached Discharge List with patient predischarge.	.75 hours

Exhibit 1.11 Pain Treatment Indicator Example

Care or Service Outcome Indicators	Performance or Process Indicators	Financial Indicators
Care (clinical and satisfaction) or service results	Recommended process and employee responsibilities	Necessary or avoidable cost

Strategic Priority: *Improve and expand pain management and treatment program.*
Performance Improvement Priority: *Improve orientation to pain treatment for patients and their families while decreasing costs.*

Care or Service Outcome Indicators	Performance or Process Indicators	Financial Indicators
Productivity Management Maintain full-time equivalent (FTE) budget at ± 2% of target (adjusted for volume).	1. Track and trend volume and acuity levels daily, by shift.	.25 hours
	2. As budgeted positions are vacated, fill only those that are volume and acuity justified.	0–3 hours
	3. Preschedule, based on anticipated volume and acuity.	2.0 hours
	4. Each shift, adjust actual staff assigned to match actual volume and acuity requirements.	1.5 hours
	5. Track and trend variations in volume and acuity to increase precision in prescheduling and justify future FTE needs.	.25 hours
	6. Submit Productivity Report with a brief narrative explaining variances, at the end of the pay period.	1.0 hours
		Total = 5–8 hours per pay period

Indicator Development Worksheet

Exhibit 1.12 Manager Performance Indicator

Strategic Priority: *Cost containment*
Performance Improvement Priority: *Patient and employee safety*

Care or Service Outcome Indicators Care (clinical and satisfaction) or service results	Performance or Process Indicators Recommended process and employee responsibilities	Financial Indicators Necessary or avoidable cost
LABOR WORKERS DISABILITY Employees will have no reportable injuries to OSHA (Reportable injury = missed day of work and/or given a prescription). National OSHA average is 10.*	Employees are expected to comply with all safety standards established in the organization, resulting in no reportable OSHA injuries.	Cost of employee missed days at work; cost of prescriptions paid by organization and/or employee.
INCOMPLETE MEDICAL RECORD All discharged patient's medical records will be completed by 10 days after discharge. Joint Commission standard: 50% or less of average monthly patient discharges have medical records incomplete.*	Physicians will complete their discharged patient's medical records within 10 days after discharge.	Bills cannot be submitted until medical record is complete; impacts cash flow of the organization.
EMPLOYEE NEEDLE PUNCTURES Employees will have no needle punctures.	Employees will follow all hazard waste and materials standards to prevent needle punctures.	Cost of epidemiology follow-up and treatment; cost of loss of work.
DRUG UTILIZATION REVIEW Patients will receive appropriate dose and length of Toradol® therapy.	Physicians will: - prescribe loading dose - not exceed maximum recommended daily dose (150 mg/d on Day 1; 120 mg/d thereafter) - place patient on scheduled dose or PRN regimen - indicate duration of drug therapy - use agent concomitantly with narcotic analgesic	Cost of complications due to high-risk side effects: - renal impairment - GI bleeding - nausea - Anticoagulant interaction Cost of excess use.

* Comparative standard for reference and educational purposes.

Exhibit 1.13 Assorted Cost-related Indicators

Indicator Development Worksheet

Action Section

If you are a manager, arrange a meeting with your employees. If you are not a manager, arrange a meeting with your interdisciplinary team. Using their expertise and the information from this interview process, identify the following: (1) your service's most significant outcomes (five internal and five external), ones that would convince even the most skeptical opponent that your service gives excellent care or service; (2) the process employees normally use to reliably and predictably achieve those outcomes (one process for each outcome); and (3) how much time it takes to complete each of the processes.

- Use the interview format provided (Exhibit 1.15)

- Reference the **examples** if you get stuck (Exhibits 1.8 through 1.13)

- Keep the **Quick Guide** close by to help you (Exhibit 1.14)

- Document the output from the group on the blank **Indicator Development Worksheet** (Exhibit 1.16).

Quick Guide (Cheat Sheet) for Developing Indicators

Care or Service Outcome Indicators Care (clinical and satisfaction) or service results	Performance or Process Indicators Recommended process and employee responsibilities	Financial Indicators Necessary or avoidable cost
Standards in this column identify and communicate to participating employees what is the "right thing" to do. **Indicators** in this column measure if participants have: • met the outcome • did not meet the outcome • exceeded the outcome	**Standards** in this column identify and communicate to employees how to do things the right way, the first time, using a flowchart, clinical pathway, or narrative. These **indicators** double as performance evaluation criteria to measure if participants: • met the outcome • did not meet the outcome • exceeded the outcome	These **standards** identify productivity targets and cost constraints. These **indicators** measure if productivity and financial targets have been met, not met, or exceeded.
What outcome is desired? **What goal, target, or result does the group want to achieve?** **What wish do you want to come true (be realistic)?** **What strategic and performance improvement (PI) priorities are addressed?**	**How will you achieve the desired outcome or goal?** **What is the process (to be followed) that will reliably and predictably lead to the desired results?** **What are the action steps? What should be done? What's the plan for how you will get to the target?**	**How much will it cost?** • FTE labor hours/dollars expended • Supplies and equipment

Indicator Development Worksheet

Exhibit 1.14 Indicator Development Quick Guide

Internal and External Customer Interview

Our service's key customers

What we think they want from us

_____

_____

_____

_____

_____

_____

_____

_____

_____

Directions:
After you have identified your key customers, arrange a 30-45 minute face-to-face meeting. As the supplier, use the questions below to structure your discussion. Keep in mind that customers often have unrealistic expectations, and you may need to negotiate.

1. What services, materials, or information do you need from our department? You are gathering data for the first column of the **Indicator Development Worksheet.** Probe for specifics (i.e., timeliness, effectiveness [right thing], efficiency [right way], integrity, appropriateness, etc.)?

2. How does your department use the input (services, materials, or information) our department supplies? This will help me understand your operation and how we can serve you better.

3. Are there things we're either (1) not doing or (2) not doing as well as you'd like us to do? We need this information for our department-level performance improvement planning?

Exhibit 1.15 Internal and External Customer Interview

Care or Service Outcome Indicators
Care (clinical and satisfaction) or service results

Performance or Process Indicators
Recommended process and employee responsibilities

Financial Indicators
Necessary or avoidable cost

Strategic Priority: _____

Performance Improvement Priority: _____

Indicator Development Worksheet

Exhibit 1.16 Indicator Development Worksheet

Integrated Quality Management Model

At the beginning of each section, the model shown in Figure 1.4, **Integrated Quality Management Model** is like a "you are here" map, showing both the big picture and, specifically, where you are in relation to the big picture. In addition to showing the layout of this book, it also includes the five subheadings from the Improving Organizational Performance chapter of the Joint Commission's *Accreditation Manual for Hospitals,*[5] and overlays the steps of the **10-Step Model.** The intent is for the reader to be able to align the information in this text with whatever system is currently being used within the organization. The constant is the process: planning, process design, measurement systems, assessment, and performance improvement. Each process step will be the subject of a section of the book, and, within each section, there will be tools, techniques, case studies, and information about how to achieve that step of the process. Here, like in any other process, the best processes produce the best performance.

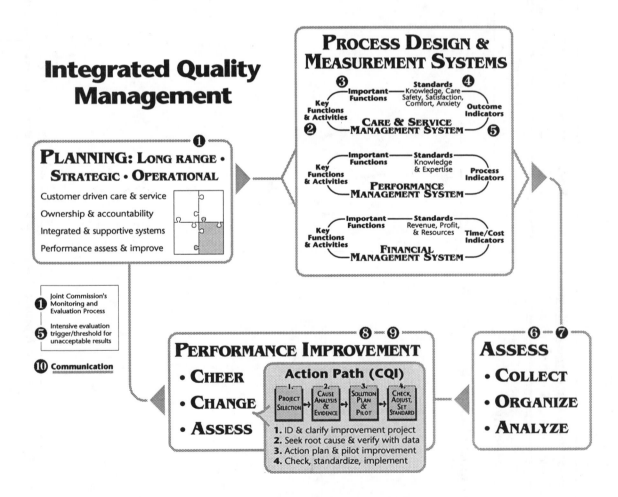

Figure 1.4 Integrated Quality Management Model

Notes

1. L.J. Peter and R. Hull, *The Peter Principle* (New York: Morrow, 1969), 159.

2. A. Kohn, *No Contest: The Case Against Competition* (Boston: Houghton Mifflin Company, 1986), 45–78.

3. R. Axelrod, *The Evolution of Cooperation* (New York: Basic Books, 1984), 173.

4. W. Byham and J. Cox, *Zapp! The Lightning of Empowerment* (New York: Harmony Books, 1990), 41.

5. Joint Commission on Accreditation of Healthcare Organizations, *Accreditation Manual for Hospitals* (Oakbrook Terrace, IL: 1996).

Recommended Reading

Beckham, D. 1995. Running with the herd: Building a business strategy. *Healthcare Forum Journal.* March–April: 62–69.

Berwick, D. 1992. Seeking systemness. *Healthcare Forum Journal.* March–April: 22–30.

Butz, H. 1995. Strategic planning: The missing link in TQM. *Quality Progress.* May: 105–108.

Coile, R. 1995. Managed care outlook 1995–2000: Top 10 trends for the HMO insurance industry. *Russ Coile's Health Trends.* March: 1, 3–8.

Fraraccio, R. 1996. Senior management commitment: The most significant driving force. *Surgical Services Management.* March: 44–45.

Joint Commission on the Accreditation of Healthcare Organizations. 1992. *Striving toward improvement: Six hospitals in search of quality.* Oakbrook Terrace, IL: Joint Commission.

Kirk, R. 1996. Maximizing quality in a managed care environment. *Surgical Services Management.* January: 35–37.

Lawrence, D., and H. Zuckerman. 1992. Strategic leadership for quality in health care. *Quality Progress.* April: 45–48.

Panel discussion: The role of quality management in healthcare today and tomorrow. 1993. *QRB/Quality Review Bulletin.* May: 158–164.

Parr, W., and C. Hild. 1995. Maintaining focus within your organization. *Quality Progress.* September: 103–106.

Rise in employer coalitions can create an attractive market for your future. 1996. *PHO Update.* February: 13–15.

Shortell, S. et al. 1995. Assessing the impact of continuous quality improvement/total quality management: Concept versus implementation. *Health Services Research.* June: 377–401.

Smith, J. et al. 1995. Using patient focus groups for a new patient services. *The Joint Commission Journal on Quality Improvement.* January: 22–31.

Smith, M. 1975. The role of CQI in the new strategic planning model for hospitals. 1994. *Strategies for Healthcare Excellence.* April: 7–12.

DESIGNING THE BEST PROCESS LEADS TO THE BEST PERFORMANCE RESULTS

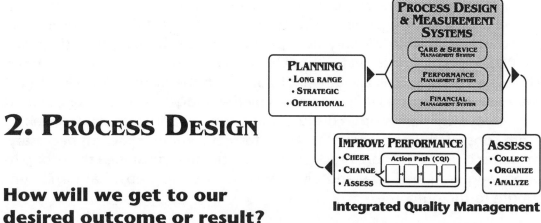

Integrated Quality Management

2. PROCESS DESIGN

How will we get to our desired outcome or result?
What process will predictably take us to target?

At one point in life, most of us have wanted to lose a pound or two... okay, maybe five. Whatever the number, it defines the desired outcome, or goal, to be achieved. The critical question becomes, "What process will reliably and predictably deliver that outcome?" Should a lock be put on the refrigerator? Should I join a gym? Should I walk 2 miles every day? What works? With some interviewing and probing of subject matter experts (people who have successfully achieved *and sustained* a 5 pound weight loss), an effective, efficient process could be, and has been, identified. The other half of the challenge is to figure out how to motivate people to follow the proven-to-be-effective process. And that's process improvement.

Patient-care processes are no different. As outlined in the previous chapter, internal and external customers must be interviewed, first, to identify, and second, to negotiate desired outcomes. Once agreed to, suppliers or providers of care must determine which process will most accurately and consistently lead to the desired outcome. If an acceptable process does not exist, subject matter experts will have to create one or study and analyze a broken process so it can be redesigned to produce a better outcome. Returning to the weight-loss example, reducing caloric intake as a stand-alone process may be insufficient. The process may need to be tweaked to include exercise, nutritional counseling, and motivational tapes—or that machine that makes nasty comments when you open the refrigerator door.

Simplifying and Streamlining Workload (a.k.a. Work Redesign, Reengineering, Process Improvement)

In 1981, as a novice consultant, I was working with a nursing division of a hospital that was under extreme cost constraints. My charge was to help them improve productivity, to do "more with less," a term that, I learned over the years, only antagonized compassionate caregivers who were already working *fast*. In fact, the key was not to do things faster, but to do less, take fewer steps, eliminate work. After this concept was reconciled, we talked about how to identify acuity-required care hours per patient day (HPPD) and how to budget for those hours based on projected patient days. Then it was time to talk about what to do when the "acuity required" HPPD were greater than the HPPD approved by the budget. As managers, should they throw their arms up in disgust, pout, whine, and complain, or take a more constructive approach? While the former sometimes seems necessary, the latter is infinitely more productive. Management must lead the group to improving workload flow and *give permission* to skip steps that don't contribute to the outcome.

Even in 1981, the issue of having sufficient time to give a desired level of care was a touchy one. Thus, the question of how to provide that level of care within constraints was a land mine waiting for a foot. As the consultant, I started talking about workload streamlining and simplification (now known as reengineering or work redesign). I pointed out that there were many processes that could be studied and streamlined. For example, the simple task of answering the phone not only interrupted caregivers but ate up their time as they traveled down a long hallway, responded to the caller, traveled back, and reoriented themselves to the task they left. I suggested that a few well-placed hall phones could be a real time saver and went on to do the related math to show dramatically how a simple change in a task could make a very big difference in time saved.

> What steps can be eliminated without compromising quality?

I was on a roll until an angry-looking nurse in the back row said, "Hey, consultant. That's easy for you to say, but this is a government hospital, and if we want a new phone, we have to go through Congress!" Boom! Stepped right on that land mine. The group groan was in harmony with her comment, and while I mentally questioned the reality of the statement, the frustration in her voice was unmistakable. This group was not only under fierce cost constraints, their level of empowerment was about minus five. At least that's how they saw it. Realizing I had lost the group's confidence, and there was no getting it back so late in the afternoon, I decided to jump ship and give them homework, which, in the end, taught us all a great deal.

The homework assignment went like this. I asked them to go back to their units and gather a few people around a flipchart for just 10 minutes of brainstorming (some worked longer, but it was their option). The brainstorming topic was, "What tasks can be done faster, in less steps, without compromising quality?" I imposed two parameters (constraints): (1) it had to be different from anything they had done before, and (2) it had to be something they could do without having to ask permission. Happily, this brought up discussion on several units as to *why* they needed permission for certain actions—an appropriate question.

The next morning, when I returned, I was happy, and surprised, to discover that my decision to jump ship was a good one. Everyone came in with their lists, and they were smiling! A couple of smart alecks wanted to know if they were going to get my fee since they came up with the answers. They didn't know I was so relieved that I would have happily given it to them. After combining and removing duplications, the final list contained 143 new ideas for streamlining and simplifying their workload. Forcing themselves to think of something different often led to a more creative answer. One unit even transferred their brainstorming to the topic of grocery shopping (How can we shop faster without compromising quality?) and then applied some of the answers to the real topic, patient care.

Too often, the process, rather than the outcome, becomes the focal point. We've got to do it this way? *Why? Who said so?* What will happen if we don't? One work redesign team from a coronary care unit (CCU) struggling to improve a process applied the "Why" technique (a sophisticated tool typically used only by 3-year-old children):

"**Why** are you doing this?"	"*Because.*"
"**Why**? For what outcome?"	"*None specifically. But we have to do it.*"
"**Why** do you have to?"	"*Because we've always done it that way.*"
"**Why** ?"	"*It's in the CCU standing orders.*"
"**Why** ?"	"*The CCU committee mandated it.*"
"**Why** did they do that?	"*Dr. X, the mean, powerful, chairman of the CCU committee, wanted it.*"
"**He's been dead 5 years.**"	"*Oh…*"

The design and analysis of processes (for the purpose of improvement) has accrued many names over the years, from *workflow analysis*, to *work redesign*, to—the current hot one—*reengineering*. Regardless of what it is called, the focus is the same: finding the best (i.e., most effective, efficient, reliable) process, one that will lead predictably to the desired outcome.

Designing Dependable, Affordable, Reimbursable Processes

For every (realistic) outcome, there is a corresponding process that will lead to its achievement. Managers have the task to identify—through discovery or design—the best process given their particular work situation and the skill level of their staff members. For them, the best process is one that is predictable (no surprises), dependable (no mistakes), and reimbursable. Achieving such an ambitious goal must be *systematized*. It's not an accident that some amusement parks are sparkling clean or that customers are delighted at one store and not another. Companies of every variety are looking at a *systems* approach to serving their customers.

Examples of different types of processes follow:

- *Standard operating procedures (payroll, dietary, laundry, needle disposal, infection control, etc.)*

- *Clinical pathways, critical paths*

- *Supply-ordering procedures*

- *The process used to dress and prepare for work*

- *Operational and capital equipment budgeting*

- *Computerized prompts: "Are you sure you want to do that? If you do, the following event(s) will occur."*

- *Customer service voice-mail queues: If you want to place an order, press 1. If you want to check an existing order, press 2. If you'd like to have more information via fax, press 3. All others, please hold (for the rest of your life).*

An example that anyone in the healthcare industry can relate to or at least knows about is the waiting time in the emergency department (ED). Those of us who have worked in hospitals with EDs know that patients are not served on a first-come-first-serve basis. The sicker the patient, the faster he or she sees the physician, usually based on a system of triage protocols that ensure consistency regardless of the time of day or staff members on duty. However, this is not common knowledge, and until a few years ago when hospitals stepped up their efforts to improve continuously, little was done to communicate this message to the public.

One ED with a huge number of complaints embarked on its process improvement efforts with a list of 70 identified problems in the ED that the team believed contributed to the long waiting times for service—a world hunger-size problem. Obviously, they could not solve all of the problems at once, so they prioritized those having the greatest impact on delays.

Initially, the team wanted to focus on streamlining all of their processes. However, the more they looked at processes, the more aware they became that many factors were simply out of their control. For example, when a lab test was ordered, they were not only at the mercy of the lab tech availability but the machinery that analyzes the blood. When a bed was vacated, time had to be taken for environmental services to clean the area. When patients arrived, they were often in clusters because emergencies aren't "scheduled" in an orderly fashion. Last, no matter how long a patient had been waiting with a broken finger, if a patient arrived later with a cardiac arrest, the "broken finger" would have to wait (unless he or she also had a cardiac arrest from the stress of hanging around the ED).

This team's first performance improvement (PI) output was *ED TV.* A closed-circuit TV was placed in the ED with information about the hospital and the standard operating procedures in the ED. Unlike the television series *ER*, the focus was on education and information rather than drama. *ED TV's* popularity, however, held its own against programmed television (on the other side of the waiting room). *ED TV* gave patients and families vital information about how the ED functioned, including priorities, procedure routines, rationale for the decisions made, and even some ideas for things to do while waiting. Simulating a real patient visit, the film walked through and explained aspects of an admission to the ED, various procedures, and both discharge and admission to the hospital.

Staff members followed through on the information sharing. While the triage nurse(s) kept patients apprised of the waiting situation, staff at the bedside kept patients and their families up-to-date with the progress of care. For example, one nurse, while participating in a "late lab results" team, learned that some tests take longer to analyze than others. She shared this new knowledge with her colleagues, and they all used it to keep patients informed, for example, "Mrs. Jones, it will take 20 to 30 minutes for the machines to calculate results. If you need to make phone calls or eat, now would be a good time, and it would give Mr. Jones an opportunity to rest a few minutes." It was an example of the power of *communication*. The more the caregivers know about concurrent processes and the needs of their current patients, the better they can negotiate a situation that will facilitate everyone's goals.

There are literally tens of thousands of processes in any given healthcare facility, and most probably contain opportunities for improvement. The processes below are frequently chosen for cross-functional teams to resolve:

Processes frequently selected as improvement opportunities

- *Medication delivery*
- *Total hip-care path*
- *Waiting time delays*
- *Purchasing*
- *Care planning*
- *Infection prevention*
- *Employee evaluation*
- *Daily staffing*

- *Admission process*
- *Staffing procedures*
- *Discharge process*
- *Tracking/trending complaints*
- *Logging/locating lost property*
- *Reporting/analyzing an injury*
- *Interviewing and hiring staff*
- *Staff orientation and training*

Flowcharts: The Key to Creating the Best Processes

By far, the easiest and most collaborative way to improve a process is to convene a group of subject matter experts—people who work with the process every day—and have them generate a flowchart. The flowchart of the "wake-up" process is a, hopefully, amusing example, but it's also one that we have all experienced, so it's a good place to start. First thing in the morning, the alarm sounds and we're faced with the first decision of the day: Should I get up? If yes, I get up. If no, I press the snooze button and go back to sleep until the alarm sounds again, presenting me with my second decision of the day: Should I get up now? Some people can stay in this "loop" all day long. Eventually, we get up and move onto the next two decisions: Is there time to eat? and Still hungry? This is another set of loops where people get stuck. In flowcharting, the goal is to identify bottlenecks, disconnects, breakdowns, and other obstacles that stand in the way of a smoothly flowing process. A smooth rendition of this example would be a straight set of actions (a standard operating procedure), whereby the alarm sounds, we get up on the first ring, eat a banana and a donut, shower, get dressed, and go to the car—without a hitch.

But that's not how it always works. One team had such a problem with tardiness that team members decided to examine their own processes for getting to work on time. After collecting data, they prioritized three root

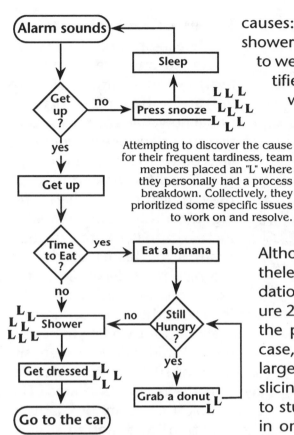

Attempting to discover the cause for their frequent tardiness, team members placed an "L" where they personally had a process breakdown. Collectively, they prioritized some specific issues to work on and resolve.

Figure 2.1 Flowchart Example

causes: (1) the snooze button, (2) long showers, and (3) inability to decide what to wear. Once the root causes were identified, they easily and quickly came up with solutions: (1) using alarm clocks without snooze buttons, (2) taking shorter (cooler) showers, and (3) selecting the next day's outfit before going to sleep. Identifying and verifying the root cause helped solve this problem.

Although this was a simple, but nonetheless real, example, it provides a foundation for the basics of flowcharting (Figure 2.1. The *oval* symbols indicate where the process begins and ends. In every case, the selected process is part of a larger process. The team or individual is slicing off one piece of a larger process to study in detail and, in fact, may zero in on an even smaller part of the process. The start/stop points remind the study group of where to focus attention and to set boundaries for the group's attention and discussion. The *square* or *rectangle* symbols indicate action and activity. Something is happening or an event is occurring. The *diamond* symbols are the decision points and are often a point at which the process breaks down or disconnects. Sometimes, wrong decisions are made, or no decision is made. Often, especially in organizations, the decision points are taken out and decided in advance to prevent error or breakdowns, and their names are changed to standard operating procedures (SOPs). Traditionally, procedures have been written in narrative; however, some organizations are getting wise and foregoing the rhetoric in favor of a visually friendly flowchart. Last, the arrows show the direction of the activity flow so that any reader can be clear about what comes next, and next, and next. Ideally, a flowchart should be simple enough to understand without explanation. A new staff member, for example, should be able to look at one, know how things are to be done, and successfully perform to the desired outcome. (See Figure 2.2.)

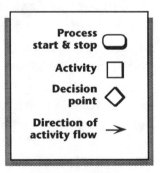

Figure 2.2 Basic Flowchart Symbols

Flowchart & Checksheet

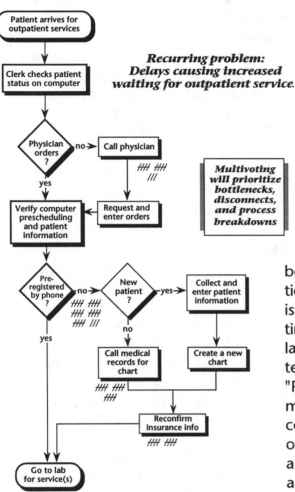

Recurring problem:
Delays causing increased
waiting for outpatient service.

Multivoting
will prioritize
bottlenecks,
disconnects,
and process
breakdowns

Figure 2.3
Outpatient Registration Flowchart

Types of Flowcharts

The "wake-up" flowchart we've discussed and the outpatient registration example (Figure 2.3) are both examples of traditional flowcharts. They are particularly useful for examining the links between activities (or functions) and for looking, first, at the big picture, and then zeroing in on the problem area(s). In the outpatient registration example, the team looked at the big picture of delays in outpatient services and identified a bottleneck at the point of registration. Patients were waiting to be registered and staff members were sitting idle while their patients were delayed in the registration area. The team took the activity box labeled "Registration" and started a new, more detailed flowchart. This process began with "Patient arrives for outpatient services," and the results are shown in Figure 2.3. This team also used multivoting to prioritize problem areas to investigate. They quickly noticed all the delays were in areas that could have been avoided altogether. Instead of focusing their attention on how to improve the on-site registration process, team members decided to work on avoiding the process altogether by making sure every possible patient was preregistered the day before. Their goal was to eliminate all of the problems that resulted when patients were not properly prescheduled and preregistered.

Matrix flowcharts are useful in looking at the relationship between different functions as well as the flow of the process as it crosses back and forth between functions. Some teams create a traditional flowchart first and then draft the matrix from that base. Adding patients or other customers such as third-party payers, also adds a new dimension to the responsibility, as they are occasionally contributors to, or root causes of, the problem. The example of the matrix flowchart in Figure 2.4 is a streamlined version of an outpatient surgical procedure that begins with the physician calling to schedule the procedure and ends with the results being reported to the patient. Initiated by a slew of patient complaints to the outpatient department, patients were primarily upset that they were not receiving their results from their physicians, something the organization had no control over once results were reported to the physician. However, as the QI coordinator probed into the issue, several problems were identified, and eventually a cross-functional team was formed to look at the procedure from start to finish.

Note there are some new symbols introduced. These are often included after the initial flowchart is created, but they help add clarity for the viewer. The *cloud* symbol is a favorite for several reasons. One, it may describe exactly how everyone in the group feels about that particular part of the process. Two, it can be used to "park" an issue temporarily until an absent team member or a knowledgeable resource can be located or to another meeting that has more agenda time available. Three, it can also be used to isolate a part of the process for which the team feels they have no control. In the example, the team initially felt they had no control over the physicians when it came to the issue of getting results from the physician to the patient; however, after discussion with the physicians (as their customer) the team implemented several new options to their process to help physicians get this information out to patients quickly and clearly.

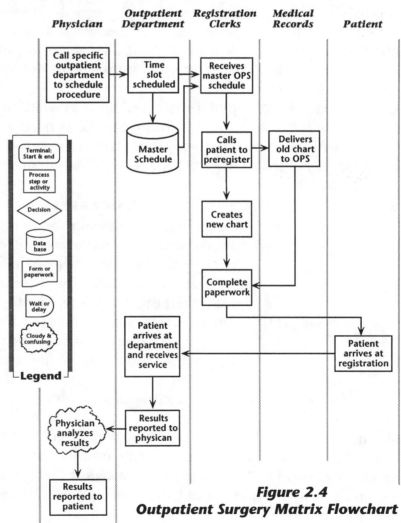

Figure 2.4
Outpatient Surgery Matrix Flowchart

Top-down flowcharts are handy for producing both a big picture, top-line look at a process as well as detail. Easiest of the flowcharts to construct, it simply follows the primary, or core, steps of the process and then provides the detail flow for each, offering the viewer both a macro and micro view of how the process flows while maintaining focus. Their value lies in their simplicity of sequence and the visual stimulation for the group to focus their attention on (1) the entire process, (2) what comes next at each step of the process, and (3) what must be done to move forward toward the end result. Top-down flowcharts are particularly useful when creating a clinical pathway that involves several different functions, all concurrently working toward their respective outcomes. (See Figure 2.5.)

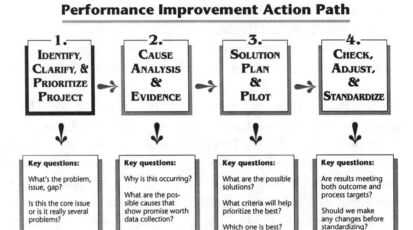

TOP-DOWN FLOWCHART
Performance Improvement Action Path

| 1. IDENTIFY, CLARIFY, & PRIORITIZE PROJECT | 2. CAUSE ANALYSIS & EVIDENCE | 3. SOLUTION PLAN & PILOT | 4. CHECK, ADJUST, & STANDARDIZE |

Key questions:

Key questions:	**Key questions:**	**Key questions:**	**Key questions:**
What's the problem, issue, gap?	Why is this occurring?	What are the possible solutions?	Are results meeting both outcome and process targets?
Is this the core issue or is it really several problems?	What are the possible causes that show promise worth data collection?	What criteria will help prioritize the best?	Should we make any changes before standardizing?
Which aspect is a customer priority?	What does the data say? Does it agree with perceptions?	Which one is best? How will we test?	How will we operationalize/implement?

Figure 2.5 Top-Down Flowchart of the Performance Improvement Action Path

Analyzing Flowcharts and Processes

Many healthcare managers are complaining (actually, pouting, whining, and complaining) that there are not enough resources—particularly the human kind—to deliver the care and service that are desirable. If you are one of those managers, accept this challenge. Identify the most time-consuming process in your department, service, or function. Pick the one you resent, the one that wastes your time or the time of your staff members. Convene your team, and streamline the process using one of these flowchart techniques.

As the team unfolds the process—looking broadly at the primary steps of the process, then zeroing in on specific problem areas—some, or all, of the questions posed in **Analyzing a Flowchart** (Exhibit 2.1) will be useful in pulling out information about the process—even when the answer is "no answer."

Analyzing a Flowchart

1.

Examine Each Decision Symbol
- Is this a checking activity?
- Is this a complete check, or do some errors go undetected?
- Is this a redundant check?

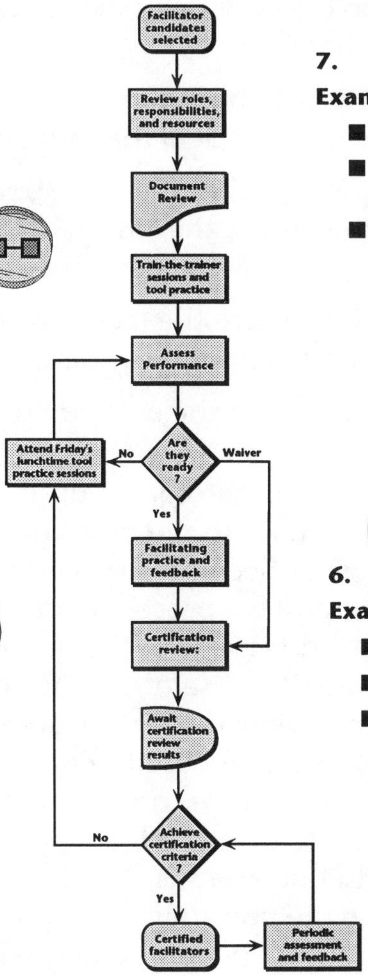

2.

Examine Each Rework Loop
- Would we need to perform these activities if we had no failures?
- How "long" is this rework loop (steps, time lost, resources consumed, etc.)?
- Does this rework loop prevent the problem from recurring?

3.

Examine Each Activity Symbol
- Is this a redundant activity?
- What is the value of this activity relative to its cost?
- How have we prevented errors in this activity?

4.

Examine Each Document or Database Symbol
- Is this necessary?
- How is it kept up-to-date?
- Is there a single source for the information?
- How can we use this information to monitor and improve the process?

7.

Examine Overall Flow
- Is the flow logical?
- Are there any "leaks" or "black holes"?
- Are there parallel tracks or multiple pathways, and, if so, is the rationale sound?

6.

Examine Each Handoff
- Who is involved?
- What could go wrong?
- Are suppliers meeting the customer's needs? How?

5.

Examine Each Wait Symbol
- What are we waiting for?
- What complexities does this wait give rise to?
- How long is this wait?
- How could we reduce this wait and/or its impact?

Flowchart symbols (center):
- Facilitator candidates selected
- Review roles, responsibilities, and resources
- Document Review
- Train-the-trainer sessions and tool practice
- Assess Performance
- Are they ready? → No → Attend Friday's lunchtime tool practice sessions; Waiver; Yes
- Facilitating practice and feedback
- Certification review
- Await certification review results
- Achieve certification criteria? → No; Yes
- Certified facilitators
- Periodic assessment and feedback

Exhibit 2.1 Analyzing a Flowchart

Reproduced, with permission, from the syllabus, *Methods and Tools of Quality Improvement,* originally developed by Paul E. Plsek & Shan Cretin, and copyrighted by the Institute for Healthcare Improvement. © 1994 Institute for Healthcare Improvement.

Here is some additional flowcharting information:

- **Decision** points (diamonds) - These often cause delays, because of excess checking activities and indecision.

- **Rework** loops - Whole departments have been created to deal with a path of rework that could have been prevented.

- **Activities** - Too often, activities are accepted as is because "we've always done it that way."

- **Document and databases** - Many functions, even organizations are drowning in a sea of data that are not necessarily informative.

- **Wait symbol** - If a patient is asked about his or her hospital stay or outpatient procedure, the length of the waiting time (positive or negative) will most likely be mentioned.

- **Handoffs** - This is where the race is won or lost. The interface between departments cannot be underestimated.

- **Overall** - Does it deliver the desired outcome or not?

Turf is a recurring theme that comes up during most of the above-mentioned aspects of flowcharting. It comes up because members of different turf ~~gangs~~ groups try to become a unified team with the responsibility to resolve an issue or improve a process. Participants of relay races know that many races are won, and lost, with the handoff. The same theory holds for providing patient care. Because of the lack of control or influence departments and functions have had over one another in the past, they've pulled tightly into themselves and focused only on what they could control. As a result, a great admitting office, great lab, and great nursing unit, collectively, may not be able to do a great job for the patient because of the handoff, or interface, with one another. Much of the success of teams has been related to smoothing the transition from one function to another, removing duplication of their work, and integrating services they provide.

A case study. The standard procedure for processing a physician's order was being reviewed by a clinical path team. One big bottleneck was the unit secretary's typically time-consuming hunt for a registered nurse (RN) to check the transcribed orders. Questions were raised by the team. Why must the RN sign off the order? The order is always checked by the receiving department (pharmacy, lab, radiology, etc.) before being carried out. Were the hassles and delays—locating the nurse and processing the order—worth it in terms of clinical outcome? The team goal was to eliminate steps without compromising the quality of their outcomes, and that's exactly what they did. In the new, shorter process unit secretaries were accountable for

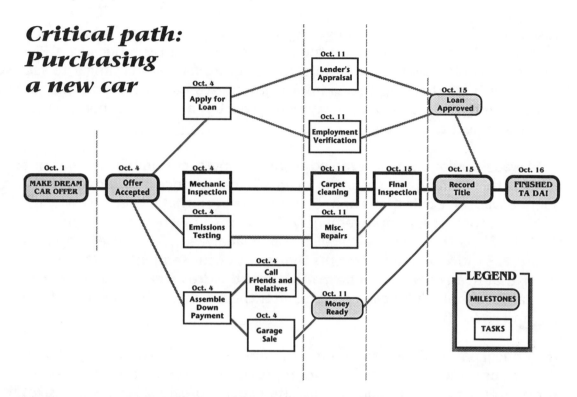

Critical path:
Purchasing
a new car

Figure 2.6 Critical Path Method (CPM) Example

transcribing and forwarding orders to the appropriate departments; the results were impressive. The unit secretaries gained time because they didn't have to locate an RN every time they had to take off an order. The RNs gained time and had fewer interruptions. Data collection documented fewer transcription errors after the unit secretaries became solely responsible for this task. A success story: fewer steps without compromising quality outcomes.

Clinical Paths Lead to Cost-Effective Results

Clinical pathways have many different names: Critical paths, practice guidelines/parameters, clinical guidelines, and clinical protocols/algorithms, to name a few. Regardless of the name, the intent is the same: (1) to assemble caregivers who contribute to a given diagnosis or procedure and (2) use their expertise to design a plan of care that is effective, coordinated, and streamlined to be efficient. Their acceptance has grown widely as more and more data confirm and document cost reductions while at the same time, clinical outcomes are maintained and, often, improved.

The concept is a derivative of the critical path method (CPM), a technique developed by engineers at the Du Pont Company in the 1950s for planning and control purposes. Using a familiar example, Figure 2.6 shows both a series of tasks and the milestones to which they lead. The critical path is the *shortest possible route from project start to project end.* In the healthcare industry, the "project" can be anything from a chest x-ray to a total knee replacement. The complexity of the process is not an issue because CPM breaks the project down into simple, more controllable parts similar to scientific methods used in process improvement. It's easier, for example, to focus on and analyze the down payment aspect of a purchase than to analyze the project as a whole.

CPM was popular because it forced planning and accountability. It was not applied to planning for recurring events because once the repetitive sequence was set, control was unnecessary. However, that is precisely why it's so helpful to process improvement. After teams flowchart a core process, the critical path should be calculated and analyzed. The car example in Figure 2.6 shows a series of events that must occur sequentially (bold outlines), that is, an offer cannot be made before the dream car has been found, the carpet shouldn't be cleaned until after the mechanic has inspected the car, and so forth.

The critical path is important to process improvement teams because it provides opportunity for breakthrough improvements by focusing the team's attention on common goals. Teams often spend precious (and expensive) time improving and streamlining activities that have little impact on im-

---

Clinical Path Definitions

Critical (clinical) pathway
Multidisciplinary **action planning**, by process owners and stakeholders, to design processes that will reliably and predictably deliver on **desired** clinical **outcomes** at the **lowest** possible **cost**. The process map shows interventions or processes used to deliver care. Recording takes place on the actual map, which becomes part of the medical record.

Variances
Displays the degree of variation from the pathway. When the variance is unacceptable over a period of time, the team can apply the scientific method to reduce the variation in the process itself. Possible causes:

- Patient or family: Refusals, complications, improvements, scheduling issues
- Clinician: Physician decision or care plan revision
- System: Lack of bed, equipment down, incomplete evaluation, or missing test results
- Community: Shortage of selected professionals, over supply of beds, reputation

Case manager
A clinical professional (usually, but not always, a nurse) who is responsible for coordinating all aspects of the patient's care plan, including monitoring and evaluation of the patient's progression along and variance from the critical path.

Clinical Path Overview

What - Interdisciplinary **action planning** to design processes that will reliably and predictably deliver on **desired** clinical **outcomes** at the **lowest** possible **cost**.

Who - **Process owners** and stakeholders.

How - Identify a **process**, diagnosis-related group (DRG), or care path to **study** in detail.

- Assemble subject matter **experts**.

- **Flowchart** existing patterns of care for medications, consultations, activities, tests and treatments, nutrition, teaching, protocols, and discharge. Understand causes of variation.

- **Study** and **evaluate** patterns of care, bottlenecks, and breakdowns.

- **Create, repair, redesign, streamline** process, develop outcome/process measures.

- **Plan** for implementation, communicate, and pilot.

- Check results, adjust, **standardize**, monitor.

Exhibit 2.2 Clinical Path Information

proving the overall flow, efficiency, or outcomes. The best way for any process to be improved is to analyze and streamline activities along the critical path. The *effectiveness* of the activities along the critical path will determine the capability of the process to achieve clinical and financial outcomes. The *efficiency* and *volume* of activities along the critical path will determine the cost in terms of time and resources.

CPM can help clinical path teams. (See Exhibit 2.2.) As clinical functions merge their individual flowcharts, displaying how they deliver care, there will be some activities that have to be accomplished sequentially, creating a critical path through the patient's course of care. Analysis by subject matter experts will distinguish those activities and milestones from those that have slack time available. To make a significant change in the outcome or efficiency of a process, the team must focus on the activities occurring along the critical path. In the critical path of a total knee replacement, for example, the postop exercise cannot begin until *after* the surgery is completed, but extensive preadmission education has contributed to shortening the length of stay and reducing resource costs overall.

More and more providers are reengineering, or redesigning, their clinical processes into streamlined, integrated, and conflict-free clinical paths with the capacity to accommodate and respond to the following:

- Who is our population?
- What outcomes do we want to achieve?
- What process will achieve outcomes most cost-efficiently?
- What resources do we need?
- How does the process flow? What does it (really) look like?
- How should the process flow? What should it (ideally) look like?

Teams with mastery of flowcharting skills have an advantage when it comes to creating clinical paths because analyzing process flow is at the core of every path. In fact, team members frequently create independent flowcharts and then combine them to reach agreement on the broad process. This method has proven effective for both resolving disagreements about the process flow and constructing a process from scratch. Creating top-down flowcharts for each day of a patient's stay, for example, allows the case to be looked at as a whole. Sibley Memorial Hospital, featured in Exhibits 2.3 and 2.4, used this approach. When the team started working on this path, the length of stay was 10 days. Over a period of 2 years and a lot of work by the team, the path got shorter and shorter (the latest version, Exhibit 2.4, is 4 days), and the outcomes got better and better. Among other things, they discovered several disciplines wanted to work with the patient at the same time, causing scheduling problems.

SIBLEY MEMORIAL HOSPITAL

TREATMENT PATH FOR PRIMARY ELECTIVE TOTAL HIP REPLACEMENT PATIENTS

	PREADMISSION	Hospital Day #1	Hospital Day #2	Hospital Day #3	Hospital Day #4	Hospital Day #5	Hospital Day #6
CONSULTS		Holding area, 2W, OR, PACU	Social Service				
TESTS - CBC, Chem 7, H & H, PT/PTT, T + X, Pre-Hip, Urinalysis, EKG, Chest X-ray, Blood Donation, Replacement X-ray		Order for OT/PT Post Hip Replacement X-ray	Hct/Hgb PT	Hct/Hgb PT	Hct/Hgb PT	PT	PT
ACTIVITY		Abduction/wedge, sling tx, bedrest, tilts/turns	Dangle/pivot, OOB to chair, ankle pumps, start PT/OT	Use of leg lifter, stand with walker	Leg lifter, stand with walker	Use walker, ambulate, use bathroom	Ambulate
TREATMENT		Hemovac, IV, Venodynes, I&O	Hemovac, Hep Loc/IV, Venodynes, Foley?	Hep Loc, BSC, D/C Venodynes and Foley	Dressing chg, BSC, D/C Hemovac		D/C Hep Loc
DIET		As tolerated	As tolerated, push fluids	Regular or as ordered	Regular or as ordered	Regular or as ordered	Regular or as ordered
MEDICATION		IM-prn, PCA IV antibiotics, home meds con't, anticoagulant	IM-prn, PCA IV antibiotics, anticoagulant	IM/PCA transition to PO prn, Loc, D/C IV antibiotic, anticoagulant	PO pain meds, LOC, anticoagulant	PO pain meds anticoagulant	Rx on chart for home pain meds, D/C anticoagulant
TEACHING		I/S, pressure areas	I/S, pressure areas leg lifter, total hip precautions	I/S, position changes	I/S	I/S	I/S, home prep, meds, hip precaution, follow-up appt.
DISCHARGE PLANNING				Introduce SW, discuss options, contact family, if needed	Rediscuss options with patient/family, make referrals, if appropriate, check insurance	Get patient preferences, make referrals, order equipment	Finalize discharge arrangements
ACTIVITIES/PREOP • Begin teaching ambulation in parallel bars > walkers > crutches • Wt. bearing • Stairs		Surgery		Begin ambulation	Increasing distances (therapy bid days 3 to discharge), stairs		
Exercises Quad sets, glut sets, ankle pumps, heel glides, SAG, sidelying/abduction prone/upper extremity *Explain exercises*			Begin quad sets, glut sets, ankle pumps	Add heel slides, SAQ	Continue exercises (days 4–6), home exercise program, sidelying Abd, prone extension per physician preference		Begin quad sets, glut sets, ankle pumps
Transfers Toilet, bed, tub, car *Review treatments*			Bed > chair transfers	Toilet transfers			
O.T. Evaluation dressings Transfers precautions *Introduce precautions assistive devices*			OT Assessment		1 hour OT session, dressing treatment precautions		Review sessions

Exhibit 2.3 Treatment Path: Total Hip Replacement
Contributed by: Joan Vincent, RN, MSN, MS, Director of Education and Training • Sibley Memorial Hospital. For reference only.

SIBLEY MEMORIAL HOSPITAL

TREATMENT PATH FOR PRIMARY ELECTIVE TOTAL HIP REPLACEMENT PATIENTS

	PREADMISSION	Hospital Day #1	Hospital Day #2	Hospital Day #3	Hospital Day #4 To Discharge
CONSULTS	Social Service evaluation (per physician preference)	Holding area, 2W, OR, PACU		Social Service	
TESTS	CBC, Chem 7, PT/PTT, T & S, urinalysis, EKG, chest X-ray, blood donation, and pre-hip replacement X-ray	Post-hip replacement X-ray	Hct, Hgb PT	Hct/Hgb PT	Hct/Hgb PT
ACTIVITY	*Hip Education Class* Begin teaching ambulation > walkers > crutches, wt. bearing, stairs	Surgery, order for OT/PT, abduction wedge/sling tx., bedrest, tilts/turns	Start PT/OT dangle/pivot begin ambulation	PT BID Use leg lifter, continue ambulation increase distance	PT BID Continue ambulation; increase distance, stairs, walker bathroom
Exercises	Quad sets, glute sets, ankle pumps, heel slides, SAQ, Upper extremity exercises *Explain Exercises*		Ankle pumps quad sets, glute sets, upper extremity exercises	Add heel slides/SAQ Begin teaching home exercise program	Continue exercises *Add: sidelying abduction, prone extension (per physician order)*
Transfers	Toilet, bed, car *Review treatments*		OOB to chair	Transfer to toilet	
Occupational Therapy	Evaluation dressings Transfers precautions *Introduce precautions, assistive devices*		OT assessment Hip precautions		One-hour OT session Dressing, treatments, precautions Car transfers
TREATMENT		Hemovac, IV Venodynes, I & O	Hemovac, Hep Lock/IV, Teds, Venodynes, Foley, I & O	Hep Lock, BSC, D/C Venodynes, Foley, Hemovac	D/C Teds Dressing change, BSC D/C Hep Lock
DIET		As tolerated	As tolerated, push fluids	Regular or as ordered	Regular or as ordered
MEDICATION		IM-PRN/PCA, IV antibiotics, home meds con't., anticoagulant	IM-PRN/PCA, IV antibiotics, anticoagulant	IM/PCA transition to PO PRN, D/C IV antibiotics, anticoagulant, laxative	Rx on chart for home meds: antibiotics, pain meds, laxative D/C anticoagulant
TEACHING	Hip education class	I/S, pressure areas	I/S, pressure areas Leg lifter Total hip precautions	I/S, pressure areas Leg lifter	I/S home prep, meds, hip precaution Follow-up appt.
VARIANCES					

Exhibit 2.4 *Treatment Path: Total Hip Replacement*
Contributed by: *Joan Vincent, RN, MSN, MS, Director of Education and Training • Sibley Memorial Hospital. For reference only.*

After discovery, some of the workload was reallocated, scheduling hassles were greatly reduced, and redundancies were removed. When a group of knowledgeable staff members makes the time to study an issue objectively and analyze each step of the process, their time spent is almost always productive. Almost...

Have you ever been in a meeting where you thought everyone had reached consensus, but after the meeting, walking down the hall, you hear someone say, "I'm not doing that!" *Consensus is not just agreeing. It's a personal commitment to change the way you do something.* There is an accountability for the subject matter experts analyzing a clinical pathway to present their knowledge and data to the team so that the best possible decisions can be made on behalf of the patient. It means physicians and all professionals involved in the care of the patient agree—unless it is inappropriate for a particular patient—to change their practice patterns and processes and adhere to the accepted process, or pathway. Many hospitals are struggling with this accountability because key professionals did not participate in the creation of the pathway. Learn from their mistakes and involve key players, especially physicians, from the very first flowchart of the process.

	Advantages	Disadvantages	Use when:
Flow-charting how the process REALLY flows	A visual of the actual process makes it easier for the team to see and address problem areas. Enables both team members and others to provide input and prioritize breakdowns, disconnects, and bottlenecks. Identifies *possible* root causes, pinpointing data collection sites. Useful war stories.	Teams have a tendency to get bogged down in details first, rather than looking at the process as a whole. Heated arguments and conflicts often ensue, which are tricky to facilitate. Occasionally, the war stories turn into whiny gripe sessions without data to verify claims and comments.	The team takes its first look at the process. It's a great way to bring out major sub-issues and reconfirm membership. The team has identified a breakdown point in the process and wants to concentrate on that specific aspect.
Flow-charting how the process SHOULD flow	Anxious to fix and do things right, team members naturally gravitate to this mode. Unless it is a recurring problem, charting "how a process should flow" can lead to a quick fix. When used to create a process from scratch (design) it can quickly provide a process to study and evaluate.	The team may make a decision about the process or change the flow because of assumption rather than facts and data. Encourages the team to rush to solutions.	There is no existing process to study or fix. The team is hopelessly locked over how the process *actually* works. A temporary fix is needed to buy time to study and permanently fix the problem.

Table 2.1 Flowchart Approaches

It doesn't always matter if the team is flowcharting how they'd *like the process to perform*, or *how it actually works* (with all of its flaws). Table 2.1 describes advantages and disadvantages to each approach. Either way, the end result is usually a tighter, more reliable process or clinical path. There are several reasons for this. For one, flowcharts visually contain the group's attention to the critical path or critical steps of the process. It's much easier to stay focused on the key steps when a team leader or facilitator uses a flipchart (or Post-it™ notes) to guide a group of people through a process. Second, once the process is charted, it is usually pretty easy to see rework loops, redundant activities, and extraneous checking activities that have voluntarily attached themselves to the process over the years. Too often, instead of studying a problem and finding the root cause to repair, teams simply slap on a "Band-Aid" solution (translation: more work) and keep doing it forever, without any documentation of improvement or resolve. Each time a Band-Aid solution occurs, the process gathers complexity, creating even more opportunities to break down, disconnect, or bottleneck. Sometimes, whole departments are created to fix or respond to problems that could have been prevented altogether.

There are many stories about flowcharting and clinical path building and rebuilding that boast about streamlining the process and removing unnecessary actions; however, one of the best ways to see potential gains is to analyze your own activities for a week. Pursue the following activity to examine and streamline your own workload by using the **Personal Work Log Analysis** (Exhibit 2.5) on the following page to write down all of the activities that occupy your time during a given week. Start at the beginning of the week; make a list of activities, and each time they occur, note how much time you spent on that activity. For example, see Table 2.2.

	TIME SPENT (in Minutes)					
ACTIVITY	**M**	**T**	**W**	**TH**	**F**	**TOTALS**
Staffing and scheduling	30	30	60	20	20	160
Payroll	60	15	15	15	15	120
Staff development	45	15	60	30	30	180
Purchasing		60				60
Lost patient articles	30	30	45	15		120
Disciplinary action	60	60	60			180
Staff meeting	90					90

Table 2.2 Record of Activities for One Week

PERSONAL WORK LOG ANALYSIS

During the next week, keep a log of how you spend your time at work. In particular, log the things that take up big chunks of your time (staffing, crisis management, disciplining employees, etc.). Answer the questions for each activity and add up your total time consumed for each column.

WHAT I DID/ACTIVITY	HOW MUCH OF MY TIME WAS CONSUMED?	WAS IT THE RIGHT THING TO DO?	DID I DO IT THE RIGHT WAY? WAS THE BEST PROCESS USED?
Covered call-ins	16 hours	yes	25%
Payroll	2 hours	yes	yes
Staff development	3 hours	yes	yes
Lost charge patrol	2.5 hours	no	NA
Staff evaluations	4 hours	yes	yes
Patient care	8 hours	yes	yes
Responding to patient complaints	2.5 hours	yes	yes
Attending meetings	7 hours	yes	50%
Totals	45 hours		
Hours doing the right things the right way	27 hours	or 60%	

Exhibit 2.5 Personal Work Log Analysis Form

At the end of the week, analyze each task or activity and ask yourself: Was this useful? Was it rework? Was it redundant? Was it a checking activity? Could it have been omitted without compromising the end result? Was it the right thing to do? Did you use the best process? Put a line through the activities you determined were rework, redundant, useless, or unnecessary, and then add up how much time you spent being useful. Feel free, at any-time during the process, to add useful (and useless) activities that come to mind—as many as you can. The goal is to focus on your personal productivity and identify activities—some of which may have been assigned to you by your boss—that are compromising the effectiveness and efficiency of your own personal output.

Too often, we do things because we're afraid not to do them. More often than not, however, we are the ones in the best position to determine if that action is adding value to the process or not. If it's wasteful, it's time to stop. Otherwise, as resources become more constrained, the wasteful activities may occupy time that could be better spent in prevention or contribution to patient-care outcomes. Make it your personal goal to remove activities you've designated as rework, redundant, useless, or unnecessary.

Managed care: What is it and why should I care?

Managed care is a term that describes a system that provides healthcare at an acceptable level of quality while controlling costs. Costs are controlled by (1) negotiating preassigned (and reduced) fees for services, (2) stressing prevention, and (3) performing utilization management (pre-authorization, concurrent review, discharge planning, and complex case management). Most readers have probably heard volumes about health maintenance organizations (HMOs), preferred provider organizations (PPOs), and physician and hospital organizations (PHOs), and the impact they have had on the organization. Hospitals and other providers sign contracts with these organizations, agreeing to adhere to a set of guidelines and prices in return for receiving a certain volume of business from the managed care organization (MCO). MCOs have had a profound effect on the way patients are cared for at every level in every patient care unit. Systems designed to help staff members reliably and successfully achieve outcomes have to keep pace.

Systems that help staff members reliably and successfully achieve outcomes... what does that mean? Systems are simply a collection of processes that we all use to help us navigate through our stressful, often chaotic days at work and at home. We create systems for getting kids up, dressed, and out the door in the morning; mobilizing our staff members to complete their workload; accomplishing errands on the way home from work; some of us even have elaborate systems in place for ensuring that there's no time to exercise

---

New customers: Managed care organizations ...and what they want

- *Partnering: to advance care <u>and</u> business opportunities*

- *Access to medical record and other appropriate information:*
    - *Quality control, performance improvement, and utilization review data*
    - *Outcome studies and investigations*
    - *Discussion of data, patterns*
    - *Social worker documentation*

- *Computer interface linking databases*

- *Shared education and other meetings*

- *Face sheet accessibility*

- *Admission notification (preplanned and emergency)*

- *Accreditations*

- *Cost-effective critical paths and protocols (with documentation of outcome and cost performance)*

---

in the evening. Any of you who have worked on computers have no doubt encountered a dialog alert box that says something like "Are you sure you want to do that? If you do, ☹☹☹ ☠X☠X☠X will happen." That alert box is the software company's system for helping us follow the correct process and ensure the best outcome or results.

Some of you may be startled to hear MCOs referred to as *customers*, and yet that is precisely what they are. (Throughout this book the term MCO will include Medicare, Medicaid, HMOs, PPOs, and any other group [with a new name] that purchases healthcare for other individuals, monitors its use, and controls any part of the care regime.) Like some patients, they purchase healthcare services, only they purchase it for a group of people, sometimes gigantic groups numbering in the thousands. Their goals are pretty straight-forward. They want to buy high-quality healthcare at the lowest possible price. Their goal is to receive premiums from individuals and businesses, pay for their healthcare at a reduced or bargained rate, and then have money (profits) left over at the end of the year. It's the reduced or bargained rate part that is creating havoc for managers in healthcare organizations.

MCOs in immature markets shop primarily for the financial bargains, assuming that the organization will self-monitor to maintain high-quality levels. However, providers (hospitals, home care agencies, outpatient labs, etc.) that provide cheap prices at the cost of quality outcomes will enjoy a very brief peak in their business. In more mature markets—where managed care is old news—MCOs are looking much deeper and asking very different questions. Assuming a given price will be met they ask: How do the clinical outcomes compare? What is the customer service level? Does this provider work with us as a partner or an adversary? Do they work with us and help our staff get the information they need? What are they doing to monitor, continually improve, and sustain their performance results? The wish list on the previous page, **"New customers: Managed care organizations... and what they want,"** is an unscientific compilation of input from several MCO administrators. The ability to respond positively to these wishes may make or break a negotiation for a pending contract.

One answer to the question of why managers should care is fairly obvious. If contracts are not signed and business is not locked in, the provider organization loses out on business for the length of the contract—guaranteed. No amount of advertising or awards or accreditations can win back that business (until the next contract bid) even when the individual patient lives next door to the hospital and wants very much to have his or her care at the most convenient, high-quality provider.

Aligning Process Design with Reimbursement

Another answer is less obvious, but most managers are already aware that they have a escalating responsibility for balancing the cause and effect relationship that exists between outcomes and cost. In this book, a lot of print has been devoted to the relationship between outcome, process, and costs. In the first section, the focus was on identifying the desired outcome. In this section, the focus has been on finding the best process that will predictably and efficiently ensure the desired outcome. The question remains, will we be able to continue to provide the desired outcome with the ever-tightening available dollars allocated to providers by third-party payers (see Exhibit 2.6)? In other words, managers have to find a way to maintain, or preferably, to maximize quality outcomes in a managed care environment that is reducing available dollars and, thus, other resources. Huh?

How? Ask many managers who, while trying to manage within the constraints of reimbursement ceilings, budget cuts, and too few employees, are concerned that quality outcomes will be sacrificed for productivity and profitability targets. The following scenario may be (too) familiar. Budgeted for "x" hours of care per average modality (e.g., test, procedure, visit), the higher

Reimbursement Incentives

Indemnity

Pays for primary through after care. Reimbursement is maximized by increasing services, resources, and length of stay.

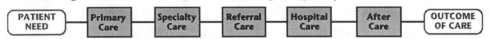

Per Diem

Pays only for hospital care. The incentive is to maximize days in hospital and minimize use of services and resources.

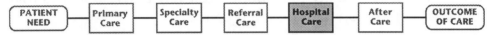

DRGs or Per-Hospital Stay*

Pays a predetermined amount for hospital and after care. The incentive is to do only what is appropriate and necessary. Length of stay, use of services, and resources are minimized.

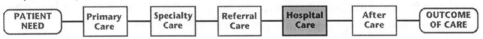

Capitation*

Pays a predetermined amount for all care related to resolving the problem. The incentive is on coordinating care, reducing resource use, and offering only necessary services in the least number of days.

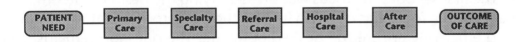

There are four primary types of third-party reimbursement (although this could change at any moment), each with their own payment plan and set of incentives for keeping down costs. Although popular in the past, per diem and indemnity plans are losing popularity to the DRG/per-hospital stay and capitated managed care (*) type plans. Capitation, in particular, will gain strength as it ultimately will give patients more choices and maintain quality while reducing paperwork, controls, and costs.

Exhibit 2.6 Reimbursement Incentives

acuity and more time-consuming modalities are all scheduled on the same day. If 2.0 care hours per modality (HPM) are needed, but the budget only provides for the average of 1.5 HPM, staff members might find themselves trying to squeeze 10 hours of care into an 8-hour day, or, equally inappropriate, taking shortcuts on care.

To avoid these kinds of responses, both cross-functional and department- or function-specific work teams need other, more acceptable alternatives and more control over how they use their time. Most important, they need reliable *methods* to help them determine and structure realistic, achievable workloads in advance. This means they need permission to let go of rituals and processes that were created by *you*. The task of accomplishing these goals while maintaining staff member satisfaction is a painstaking and delicate challenge that requires input from all who participate in the process (i.e., subject matter or content experts). The actual process of maximizing quality outcomes in a cost-constrained, managed care environment begins with the indicator development process.

Define Outcomes: Part 1 of 3

Members of all departments and functions involved in a particular plan of care must define the customer- or patient-focused clinical and service outcomes they are working to achieve. Once again, Peter's famous quote, "If you don't know where you're going, you'll probably end up somewhere else" applies.[1] Ideally, all outcomes will be aligned and compatible with one another to create an easier, more expedient, and less expensive workflow. Some outcomes will need to be negotiated, as both internal and external customers do not always have realistic, achievable expectations. Customer (e.g., patients, physicians, MCOs) requirements and preferences, however, need to be included in the outcome development process. Here's why:

- If customers have unrealistic expectations, it's far better to identify them in advance when it's easier to negotiate.

- Defining clinical and service outcomes often reveals diverse or conflicting approaches, as well as the duplication of effort.

- If patients are satisfied but the MCO is not, important business can still be lost.

- The process of defining outcomes can give everyone involved a chance to agree on what will be considered a successful outcome.

Exhibit 2.7 shows some examples of indicators. The desired patient education *outcome* (Column 1) is for patients to receive information about their condition. Specifically, and measurably, each patient will be able to verbalize certain designated information prior to his or her discharge. The next step is to create a process that will reliably deliver on that outcome.

Creating Indicators

Care or Service Outcome Indicators	Performance or Process Indicators	Financial Indicators
Care (clinical and satisfaction) or service results	Recommended process and employee responsibilities	Necessary or avoidable costs of quality

Indicator Examples

Initial assessment visit
All infants and children under the age of 1.5 years will have a Maloney evaluation completed as part of the initial assessment.

Physical therapist's responsibilities
• Complete an initial assessment that includes:
  - past medical history
  - Maloney evaluation
  - psychomotor functioning
  - current diagnosis
  - movement
  - neurological function

• Develop a plan of care and treatment based on the findings of the assessment.

1.0 Registered Physical Therapist (RPT) hour per procedure*

*1.0 Indicates the labor hours that are needed to deliver the predetermined level of care and also serves as a productivity guideline for employees.

Patient education
Standard: Each patient will receive information related to his/her condition and care of that condition.

Indicator: Each patient will verbalize, prior to discharge, knowledge of exercise, pulse, and take-home medications.

Nurse's responsibilities
Standard: The nurse will evaluate the patient's response and outcomes.

Indicator: Each nurse will document discharge knowledge status in the patient's medical record at the time of discharge.

Standard: Resources will be available and utilized appropriately.

Indicator: Individual productivity for task completion will be 30 minutes.

Exhibit 2.7 Creating Outcome, Process, and Financial Indicators

Design or Redesign Process: Part 2 of 3

Once the outcomes have been identified and clarified, the process owners (i.e., the employees who perform the process daily) play a crucial role in selecting processes that are most likely to achieve desired results efficiently and without compromising clinical or service outcomes. Some nonbelievers think this cannot be accomplished; however, case after case has shown that when teams work on improving the quality of outcomes, they also (sometimes unintentionally) reap streamlined and simplified processes. One hospital decreased a 107-step medication process to 25 steps applying the "Why" technique—questioning and challenging every step in the process—to every action and decision in its flowchart. It was an eye-opener to see how much time was spent in ritual, versus necessary, care.

When it comes to improving a process, responsibility is assigned to either a cross-functional or natural work team depending on which is best able to assess and analyze processes and improve them, when necessary, to be more effective and/or efficient. By asking probing questions like: Is the current process capable of producing the desired results? Do we really need this step? What is to be gained, or lost, if it is included or omitted? Is this a ritual or a necessity? The team can determine if the process is satisfactory, needs improvement, or needs to be discarded and redesigned or reengineered from scratch. Many quality management experts believe that if you are consistently not achieving the outcomes you want, 85% of the time it is because of the process. Either the process is ineffective and needs to be improved (or redesigned), or the process is terrific, but no one is following it. If the latter is true, accountability systems must be analyzed. Why are people not following the process? How are they being held accountable for following the process? Is the process part of their criteria-based job description, as it should be? When it comes time for the annual evaluation, are people evaluated for how many times they called in sick? More appropriately, are they being evaluated for how well they followed the process? Even better, what was their contribution to improving processes and, thus, performance results?

If staff members are faithfully following the process, however, and results are below target, it's usually an indicator that there is something wrong with the process, and it's time to study it for improvement potential. It's a worthwhile endeavor because once a process is designed —or redesigned— and accepted, it can be standardized as the *right way* to take action to achieve a particular outcome. The process may become an SOP, a clinical pathway, or a piece of a larger process. Whatever the role, the possibilities for application remain the same:

- It can be a road map for caregivers, so they not only know *what* is expected (i.e., outcome) but *how* to get there (i.e., process).

- The defined process can double as a criteria-based performance description and evaluation tool. After all, the most significant performance element that can be assessed is whether the employee is following the designated process and contributing to its ongoing improvement.

- Having a standardized process in place expedites measuring how much time the process takes to complete—an important piece of data for productivity management. Teams can even use the standard process to compare the productivity output between different skill levels.

Effectively and Efficiently Use Resources: Part 3 of 3

As processes are assessed, analyzed, and enhanced, subject matter experts must ensure that there is effective and efficient use of resources so that processes are accomplished within cost constraints. Work teams and individuals must continually ask: "If this process is followed, will we be able to stay within our time and cost constraints?" Every staff member must clearly understand that it is no longer acceptable to look only at quality outcomes; purchasers of healthcare are demanding evidence of both quality outcomes and successful cost performance.

However, the mere mention of productivity can cause staff members great anxiety. They see the faces of sick patients and worried families, wanting, needing, expecting *more* at a time when *less* is available. Some staff members assume that decreased availability of caregiver time means that patient needs cannot always be met, which is true but not necessarily detrimental. It does mean that caregivers, the subject matter experts on the process, must find significant ways to *prioritize and eliminate work that does not contribute to the desired outcome.* Working faster is not the answer. Insignificant, unrelated steps must also be eliminated to maximize efficiency. For example, a patient could be bathed *faster* by being hosed down and left to air dry, but most would consider this a (severe) compromise to patient satisfaction, comfort, and respect. A partial bath and a short back rub may be more effective to the outcome. *The reality is that healthcare providers are now living within cost constraints, and every iota of expended energy must ultimately contribute to the desired outcome.*

Knowledge of a target—how long it *should* take the care provider to complete a process—has several benefits:

- It gives employees a productivity target to work toward under normal circumstances.

- It gives managers a way to measure individual productivity performance among their employees.

- It helps identify the talented caregivers who are able to deliver care effectively and efficiently. The concept of catching someone doing something right[2] can pave the way to an improved process for all caregivers.

- When everyone is having trouble meeting the target, it is an indicator that something is wrong with the process. Data should be collected and analyzed, and a natural work team or cross-functional team should investigate.

Budgeting for Successful Performance Results

Every process that is designed comes with a cost. In this section, the discussion will move from achieving the desired results to determining if the process is affordable, and deciding what to do if it's too expensive compared to what is reimbursed. Traditionally, indicators (or measurable targets) for outcome, process, and resources have been designed into a *service unit*. The service unit is the foundation for all functional or clinical path management systems—from program and budget planning to quality and productivity monitoring and evaluation. The service unit for inpatient nursing is the *patient day* which encompasses all nursing care activities over a 24-hour period. The service unit for all other departments is generally referred to as *modality*, encompassing *procedures, tests, visits, etc.* Remarks that follow in this section will reference only modalities, for two reasons. First, a patient day is a modality that encompasses a group of interactions, activities, or tasks, and second, in the years to come, more and more patient care will be delivered (and billed) as modalities and less as patient days. Nonetheless, all methods reviewed can be used for patient days or modalities.

Also—and this is very important—a lot of attention will be paid to the individual service unit, or modality, in this section, because the more detail known about costs, the easier it is to budget for those costs, or reduce the costs, when necessary. However, the final analysis and focus are larger. We'll want to know: What is the cost of the clinical path? What is the cost of the DRG? What is the cost of running the orthopedic care unit? Thus, while budget planning may begin as a department-focused activity, it will eventually broaden as pathway teams merge care plans and redirect the focus toward a collaborative outcome. During that process, activities and tasks will be integrated, reprioritized, and even challenged, all of which may affect the budget process.

The manager's challenge is to encourage and guide staff in developing realistic, achievable outcomes (or goals) and cost-efficient processes for achieving them, so that a desired level of quality can be maintained, even enhanced, despite uncontrollable cost and availability constraints. As stated before, this does not mean "doing more with less." It means going back to the fundamentals of patient care to analyze workload in light of standards of care or desired outcomes. Are the identified outcomes realistic and achievable? Which outcomes have the highest priority? Are all tasks still necessary? Performance standards must be analyzed as well. What role does the employee play in designing and improving processes, and what accountability do they have for the results? What is the best process and what is the employee's specific contribution to patient care, service, or satisfaction outcome achievement? A manager and his or her work team should be able to

---

Measuring Employee Time Expended per Modality

Estimating
"Best guess" approach. Low cost, fast, and initially acceptable but is easily biased and doesn't always reflect current conditions.

Historical Averaging
Easy. Inexpensive. However, existing deficiencies or inefficiencies can perpetuate.

Logging
Excellent, low-cost method. Employees log activities/tasks and the actual length of time it takes to complete them (according to the predetermined performance standard). Accumulating timed activities/tasks determines total employee time involvement by modality.

Work Sampling
Experts make random, instantaneous observations and, using statistical techniques, measure the relative time spent on various work elements. The expert is usually an outside source, such as a consultant, management engineer, or industrial engineer.

Predetermined Standards
Industry-accepted standards and time studies are credible and have been scrutinized by professional leadership or have resulted from a research grant, however, individual institutions must analyze and assess applicability and acceptability of these standards.

Time & Motion Studies
A task-oriented "clipboard" and "stopwatch" approach. Each task is divided into motions that can be standardized, measured, and timed. If employees can't reach consensus on procedure or the time standard, this method can help them analyze the task/activity in more detail. It can be executed by experts or employees themselves.

Exhibit 2.8 Measuring Employee Time Expended per Modality

analyze their processes so that a *predetermined* decision of time allocation can be made for activities that consume the employees' time.

Determining standards and indicators. Do you know how much time your care (or service) and staff performance standards require? Can you afford the standard of care of 5 years ago? Analyzing the workload and determining resource time standards is one way to find out. To set and achieve realistic and compatible patient outcomes, staff performance goals, and productivity targets, managers and their staff must be able to prioritize outcomes. In other words, given their total load of responsibilities, which outcomes matter most to the customer(s)? And how much time are these outcomes consuming? Is the time spent relevant to their importance? Let's say, for example, the desired outcome is *better eating habits*. A dietitian can try to achieve the outcome by traditional, labor-consuming methods of verbally explaining and then answering questions. However, a more cost-effective, labor-saving approach might be the use of videotapes or interactive computer sessions, which would conserve the dietitian's time for comprehension assessment and clarification.

Examining tasks and activities in light of both outcome and time consumption is not new. There are many examples of streamlined, systematized processes that reduce labor time expenditure (from painting lines on the wall to guide visitors through the hospital, to direct dial phone lines, to voice mail systems, to even a system to speed the process of a patient requesting a nurse's attention). Determining accurate time allotments for tasks is an important ingredient to managing the overall workload. It's crucial to know (1) how much time a task should take, per its value and time expended, and (2) if employees can actually complete the task/activity successfully within that acceptable time frame. Some popular methods for measuring the contribution of time each employee expends per modality are reviewed in Exhibit 2.8. Each has advantages and disadvantages, so managers should select carefully, according to which will give the most credible estimate of time consumed by the activity.

At a time when professional staff want more control over their work, and acuity systems need development or revision, logging has a lot to offer. Employees have a lot of experience with the workload and can contribute positively to management decisions affecting both quality and productivity performance. Logging's focus is on developing resource time standards for all activities based on the desired outcome (standard of care) and corresponding process (performance) standards. That is, *if a target level of care is desired, corresponding labor hours must be made available, and if those hours are not available or affordable, logging data can then be used to accomplish the following*:

(1) Review desired outcomes and change expectations to something more realistic and achievable (e.g., back rubs may be limited to patients at high risk for decubitus ulcer or the interdisciplinary team priorities identified in the patient care plan).

(2) Review standards of performance and change the process or the way work is accomplished (e.g., some ED X-rays will be taken by a portable machine stored in the department, rather than transporting patients to radiology to wait or create a wait for other patients).

(3) If the above is not possible, maintain existing care and performance standards but carefully communicate identified priorities to staff, so when they don't have time to do everything, they are at least clear on what to do first.

If one of the above is not pursued, it's an automatic default to a fourth alternative: expecting the staff to make daily independent decisions about how to squeeze 10 hours of work into the 8-hour workday. The result: a combination of frustration, overtime, and unfinished work.

Logging activities help determine resource standards. The Activity Time Log, (Exhibit 2.9), is a tool to help staff members identify department standards for any task, from patient-care activities, to indirect care, to clerical functions. Some employees may initially resist getting involved—so keep it voluntary. They'll become more enthusiastic as they discover the time and patient-care benefits of determining their own standards. The logging method is affordable and simple provided you don't try to examine every single activity or task that consumes employee time. Use Pareto's 80–20 rule as a guide (i.e., 20% of the tasks studied may contribute to 80% of the quality outcomes or 80% of the time expended), and start with activities that significantly impact quality, consume the largest amount of employee time, and are considered high risk. Here's a step-by-step description of the *logging process*.

1. Staff members meet at the beginning of their shift to se-lect an activity, or task, to work on that day, and review the standards, policies, and proce-dures related to the activity. They'll decide either to follow the existing procedure or, with authorization, agree on changes *before* they begin logging their times, so that everyone will be using the same approach and the same process. Logging should include all employee time expended related to the task or activity, including indi-rect time (charting, set-up time, phone time, waiting, etc.), so processes and tasks can be analyzed for effective-ness and efficiency.

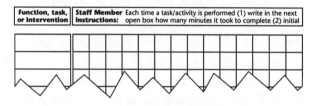

Benefits

Using this format to identify and validate time values is economical, participative, and surprisingly accurate. Staff members (1) sort through activities that are done simultaneously or in combination, (2) individually note how long it takes to do each activity, and (3) as a group, reach consensus on a target for how long it **should** *take to accomplish the activity, task, function, or intervention.*

- *Staff input/consensus: quality & productivity targets*
- *Accurate, realistic data to support acuity classification system*
- *Sharing staff skills, successes, & streamlining efforts*
- *Time study can be paced with available staff time*

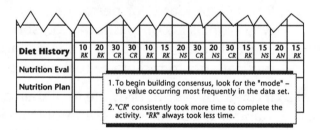

Exhibit 2.9 Activity Time Log

2. Each time staff members perform the activity, they note, on the log sheet, how long it took to complete it. At the end of the day, they meet with peers briefly to review data and their experiences. At the end of the meeting they should be able to reach agreement on specific care or service outcomes desired, the procedure or process they're going to follow, and how long it *should* take to complete (above). The next day, and every day after, they'll be able to validate, reliability test, and work toward the quality and productivity goals they agreed on that day—guided by standards to focus on the right things, following the right process. The time standard is **valid** if all appropriate actions related to the activity or task are included in the standard time and documented feedback from staff members indicates their consistent ability to complete the activity within the standard time. **Interrater reliability** is achieved when all staff members using the same processes achieve the department's standard of care for the activity or task and take the same amount of time to complete the task.

At the end of a day when several clinical or technical specialists have been focusing their expert knowledge and experience on one activity, they are usually able to agree on:

- *What the patient care outcomes should be (care standards)*

- *Specifically, what are they going to do—what processes, what accountabilities—to contribute to patient outcomes being met (performance standards)*

- *How long the activity should take in terms of their time (resource standards)*

Logging & Documenting Resource Time Standards

- Provides a log sheet of work performed
- Records volume of work completed
- Displays activities and time values

Benefits
Requires minimal training
Accounts for all time (including nonroutine)
Provides ongoing evaluation and, as needed, updating by staff
Logs and targets individual productivity
Most readily accepted by staff

Drawbacks
Disrupts work routine
Consumes staff time

---

3. How long an activity is studied depends on how quickly trends are identified and consensus is reached. Sometimes, staff members reach agreement in a few moments. Activities that can't be quickly agreed on should be studied a second, even third, day, with additional clarification of expected outcomes and processes that should be used to achieve them. Another option is to take a more in-depth look at the activity, breaking it down into parts: set-up time, waiting time, actual task time, and posttask time. Once a trend is identified and supported by data, you can move on to a new task or activity. Later, if the activity changes, or if staff members decide the assigned time no longer fits, the activity can be logged again and reevaluated.

When staff members can't reach consensus, it's usually because they're (1) using different methods or processes; (2) trying to achieve different patient care goals; (3) working with patients at different acuity levels; or (4) simply working more efficiently than others while maintaining, even maximizing, the desired level of performance outcomes. After discussion, employees are usually able to reach consensus on a process or adopt one individual's efficient, yet qualitative, way of processing the work.

4. The process of putting a time value on activities is over once employees reach agreement. Time values will have to be reviewed if the budget can't match the average *log-required* hours. However, during the logging process, efforts should remain focused on measuring the time it takes to meet targeted standards of care at a desired level of quality. Work groups naturally sift out unnecessary steps and streamline the process as they go along. It is not unusual, when the actual hours required are tallied, to discover they are more affordable than anticipated.

Some staff members try to magnify the time required for activities, but it just doesn't pay off because of the external limit to available or affordable hours and dollars. And the limit is beyond their control. When staff members are aware of time or dollar constraints ahead of time, they can use their expertise more productively by identifying ways to accomplish desired patient-care actions as effectively as possible, within the constraints. They have the best insight into which activities could be abbreviated or eliminated and how they would rank in priority.

Efficiency is doing things right,
Effectiveness is doing the right things.
And doing the wrong things less expensively
Is not much help, – Peter Drucker[3]

But the question remains: How can staff members be motivated to take such an intense interest in productivity? Financial gain? Probably not. More likely their interest will stem from the potential time gain for providing patient care safely and comfortably—so they won't feel the pressure of trying to do 10 hours of work in an 8-hour day. It makes good sense to capitalize on their expertise and instincts about quality; to look at activities in light of patient-care outcomes, performance standards, and cost; and then to use that information to maximize quality within affordable productivity margins.

Calculating the budget. Involving your own clinical or service experts in the initial logging and acuity development process is an investment that pays off far into the future. For one thing, it allows staff members to define realistic standards of care and performance, giving them more control over their workload. Second, it helps them to do their own, ongoing, interrater reliability testing by comparing time results and patient-care quality outcomes with their peers. Their involvement leads to ownership and commitment to those time standards that will ultimately determine daily staffing. Third, validity testing of time values will be ongoing—each time employees perform a modality, they can compare their knowledge of how long it *should* take with how long it *actually* takes and note factors that made the difference. The difference may be due to their own productivity, a new or infrequently used procedure, a difficult patient, or a breakdown of a piece of equipment. Whatever the reason, their knowledge of the interference, combined with their knowledge of *how it should be done,* is the best route to resolution.

Calculating Standards
Using Retrospective Classification Data

Department or Service Line Modalities	Modalities Completed & Charged		Required Hours per Modality*		Staff Hours Required
Modality # 1	1,000	X	.5	=	500
Modality # 2	1,000	X	.7	=	700
Modality # 3	1,000	X	1.0	=	1,000
Modality # 4	1,000	X	1.3	=	1,300
Modality # 5	1,000	X	1.5	=	1,500
Modality # 6	1,000	X	2.0	=	2,000
Totals	**6,000**				**7,000**

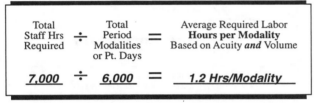

Total Staff Hrs Required	÷	Total Period Modalities or Pt. Days	=	Average Required Labor **Hours per Modality** Based on Acuity *and* Volume
7,000	÷	**6,000**	=	**1.2 Hrs/Modality**

*Hours reflect direct, "hands-on" care from logging activities. They exclude fixed (manager, clerks) and nonproductive hours paid for sick, vacation, etc.

Exhibit 2.10 Calculating Standards Form

Last, but very important, after standard activity times are validated and deemed reliable, they can be used to generate an acuity-based (flexible) operating budget. As acuity-required hours accumulate over time, they provide a numerical profile of the average patient acuity and care requirements. An example of annual accumulation is shown in Exhibit 2.10. When the required HPM (0.5 HPM, 1.0 HPM, etc.) are accumulated and averaged, they create 1.2 acuity-required HPM, the focal point of all departmental financial and quality planning. Departments with minimal variation in the time it takes to complete their units of service—a critical care unit with patients who are all critical and all require 12 hours of care per patient day or a physical therapy department, where most modalities take 30 to 45 minutes—also have less variation, on a daily basis, because of the acuity of their workload.

Remember, the goal of budgeting is to plan in advance for the resources that will be needed on a daily basis. *If both the average hours needed per modality and the number of modalities expected are identified,* a flexible human resource budget can be calculated as well as a staffing plan for the entire fiscal year.

The process begins with calculating annual full-time equivalents (FTEs). Keep in mind that 1.0 FTE may be one full-time employee working 5 days per week or several people working part-time to complete the five days (e.g., five people working one day per week each). In Exhibit 2.11, the top example shows how to calculate re-

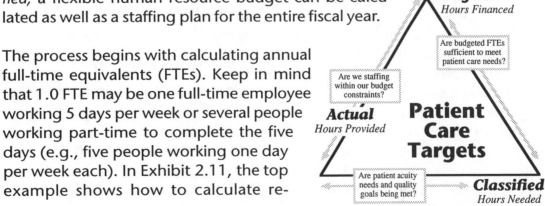

quired annual FTEs, based on the accumulated average acuity-required, and the desired 1.2 HPM. However, the calculation on the bottom shows a reality most readers will recognize: a 1.0 reduction in the FTE budget, from 8.4 to 7.4 FTEs. Most of us have experienced the disappointment of a budget cut, but even in a mandate, there is usually some choice about where the cut is made. We can cut the fixed FTE (the clerks, clinicians, managers) or the nonproductive benefit hours (if we have a death wish) or, last, the HPM. Most managers initially opt to cut the fixed FTE, in particular, manager hours, because it's fast, easy, and doesn't take away from patient care, at least not on paper.

Managers would do better to base their decision on the workload and the impact of the workload on patient-care outcomes. For example, if a manager has used the activity logs for his or her own workload and has documented 40 hours of justified management responsibilities per week, it would be foolish to reduce the 1.0 FTE budgeted for the manager. That manager would continually end up shifting his or her patient assignment to employees and creating an overload that could affect quality significantly. When this is the case, it's usually better to take out the 40 hours per

---

Calculating Annual FTEs

Using an Acuity Weighted Standard Hours per Patient Day (HPPD)

	1.2	Acuity Weighted & Budget HPM*
x	**10,000**	Projected Annual Modalities*
=	**12,000**	Annual Direct Hours Needed
÷	**2080**	Annual Hours Worked per FTE*
=	**5.8**	Direct FTEs
+	**0.6**	Nonproductive (NP) FTE†
=	**6.4**	Flexible FTEs
+	**2.0**	Fixed FTEs
=	**8.4**	**Total Annual FTEs**

* Given information.
† 24.0 (Direct FTEs) x 232 (annual benefit hrs per FTE) ÷ 2080 = 2.7 or 27.0 (Direct + Fixed) x 232 ÷ 2080 = 3.0 NP FTEs.

Calculating the Impact

of a **1.0 Reduction** in the Approved FTE Budget

	7.4	Total Available FTEs*
–	**2.0**	Fixed FTEs*
=	**5.4**	Flexible FTEs
–	**0.6**	Nonproductive (NP) FTEs*†
=	**4.8**	Direct FTEs
x	**2080**	Annual Hours Worked per FTE*
=	**9,984**	Annual Direct Care Hours
÷	**10,000**	Projected Modalities*
=	**1.0**	**Available/Budget HPM**

* Given information.
† Note: NP FTE (above) is given, not calculated.

Exhibit 2.11 Budget Calculation

week (1.0 FTE) on an annual, rather than a daily, basis. That way, on the average, it will only affect each modality .2 hours, or 12 minutes. Employees, themselves, looking back at time logs, can determine whether or not 12 minutes can be carved out of their workload in one of these ways:

- by changing the process and eliminating steps and work, without compromising quality (computers, cross-training, work simplification ideas)

- by changing standards of care to targets that are more realistic and achievable

- by identifying low-priority activities to *as-needed* or *as-ordered* status

If average acuity-required hours are 1.2 HPM, but the budget is only 1.0, and you can only staff enough to provide 0.8, something has to give, besides the staff members. Whatever the changes, once they are agreed to, they must be merged into and reflected by the acuity-based staffing plan. Make the decision proactively, plan for it, and give employees guidelines for decision making. They need to have permission to have a reasonable, achievable workload, and it should be determined in advance, ideally, by the employees. When the employees are armed with this information and knowledge of their workload, they are more aware of their individual time as it relates to patient care. They can do mini cost-benefit analyses about the patient care tasks and activities (e.g., are the patient outcomes worth the expenditure of my time as it relates to the hours available?). Further, they can make intelligent, well-informed, proactive decisions about which activities have the most significant impact on quality and are most important to retain in their daily routines.

The pressure is on every healthcare manager to cut positions, increase productivity, and do more with less. However, there are some limits to productivity improvements, and the burden of safe care weighs heavily on those who have to make the decision of what to leave out or what to do faster. Those answers should not be left to the employee working 3 to 11 Friday night who's working short staffed to cover an absence. Managers and employees must know and be able to validate (1) what they want to do for the patient at a predetermined, and mutually agreed on, level of quality; (2) the process they will use to achieve that goal in the most efficient way; and (3) how long it should take for competent staff to complete the task at the target quality level. By taking the time and effort to achieve these objectives, managers can plan their departmental workloads for maximum quality and financial benefit rather than hold their breath hoping everything will be okay. If healthcare managers do not take charge of this responsibility, someone else will gladly do it for them, but they may not have patients', or employees' best interests at heart.

Marketing to Managed Care Organizations

In the final analysis, if a manager can manage outcomes (via a well-designed, cost-efficient process), then he or she will be able to compete in the managed care marketplace.

Managing outcomes = Managing managed care

- *Use customer feedback to target, negotiate, and prioritize clinical and customer service outcomes.*

- *Design (reengineer) cost-effective, efficient processes that consistently produce desired performance results within cost constraints set by MCOs and other purchasers.*

- *Hold staff members accountable for adhering to process or improving the process when necessary.*

- *Measure, improve, document, sustain, and communicate performance results.*

One healthcare system, comprised of several rehabilitation facilities, successfully applied the above processes and easily won the managed care contracts of its choice. After identifying the top 10 procedures (total hip, total knee, etc.), process owners created clinical paths for each. Each clinical path also included (1) admission criteria, (2) discharge criteria, (3) a list of clinical outcomes to be achieved, and (4) a price tag. In effect, they were creating their own DRG or capitated system. There was a target number of days in the clinical path, but the discharge criteria and clinical outcomes drove the length of stay, not the clinical path. If a patient needed more resources than anticipated, the system absorbed the extra costs. If a patient needed less, more profit became available. The MCO loved it (actually the medical director was gushing), because it knew exactly what it was getting into as it related to cost.

Organizations, departments, and functions that have (1) identified the outcomes that need to be achieved, (2) created processes that can deliver on the outcomes, in a (3) cost-effective, cost-efficient manner—without compromising clinical and service outcomes—will definitely have the edge in surviving the financially challenged years ahead.

Notes

1. L.J. Peter and R. Hull, *The Peter Principle* (New York: Morrow, 1969), 159.

2. K.H. Blanchard and S. Johnson, *The One Minute Manager* (New York: Morrow, 1982).

3. P. Drucker, *Management: Tasks, Responsibilities, Practices* (New York: Harper & Row, 1973).

Recommended Reading

Activity-based cost system eliminates the money guessing game. 1996. *Hospital Case Management.* April: 49–53.

Bartling, A. 1995. Trends in managed care. *Healthcare Executive.* March/April: 6–11.

Bergman, R. 1994. Getting the goods on guidelines. *Hospitals & Health Networks.* October 20: 70–74.

Berwick, D. 1996. The year of "how": New systems for delivering healthcare. *Quality Connections.* Winter: 1–4.

Bonastia, C. 1994. All guidelines are not created equal. *Outcomes Measurement and Management.* September–October: 3–5.

Coffee, R. et al. 1992. An introduction to critical paths. *Quality Management in Health Care.* Fall: 1–8.

Demott, K. 1994. Critical pathways save $6.4M, cut ALOS at The Christ Hospital. *Report on Medical Guidelines & Outcomes Research.* September 22: 1–2, 5.

Fraser, I. et.al. 1993. Managed care: Where will your hospital fit it? *Hospitals.* April 5: 18–25.

Goldratt, E. 1986. *The goal: A process of ongoing improvement.* Croton-on-Hudson, NY: North River Press.

Kennedy, M. 1995. Ten strategies for masking clinical guidelines and pathways work. *The Quality Letter for Healthcare Leaders.* October: 2–12.

Lumsdon, K., and M. Hagland. 1993. Mapping care. *Hospitals & Health Networks.* October 20: 34–40.

Pehrson, G. 1994. Using care process models to improve quality while controlling cost. *The Quality Letter for Healthcare Leaders.* April: 24–27.

Rauber, C. 1995. A system that tries harder. *Healthcare Forum Journal.* November/December: 32–34.

Rupp, R., and J. Russell. 1994. The golden rules of process redesign. *Quality Progress.* December: 85–90.

Schriefer, J. 1995. Managing critical pathway variances. *Quality Management in Health Care.* Winter: 30–42.

Schriefer, J. et al. 1996. Linking process improvement, critical paths, and outcome data to increased profitability. *Surgical Services Management.* June: 46–50.

Woodyard, L., and J. Sheetz. 1993. Critical pathway patient outcomes: The missing standard. *Journal of Nursing Care Quality.* October: 51–57.

IF YOU CAN'T MEASURE IT, YOU CAN'T MANAGE IT

- ANONYMOUS

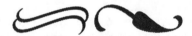

IF YOU DON'T MEASURE IT, IT WON'T HAPPEN

- ANONYMOUS

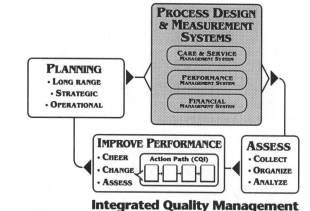

Integrated Quality Management

3. Measurement

Why is measurement suddenly so important?

It's safe to assume that most people who work in the healthcare field do not want to give up their "day jobs" to collect data. In fact, many of us who went into healthcare did so because we were people oriented and didn't want to get stuck working with all those numbers. Some might have burned college statistics textbooks, thinking, "I'll never use that again." I burned three, from three different courses, and if someone had told me that I would be yearning for those (already highlighted and underlined) texts, I would have suggested they get counseling. It's easy to measure the healthcare community's feelings about data by just mentioning the subject. Eyes roll, blink, wince, and glaze over. Some are just plain allergic to numbers. Others just don't like to be measured. With measurement comes accountability and a fear that the numbers won't show the reality. But that is precisely why good, solid, reliable data are so important to all of our futures.

Picture this scenario. Mike Wallace of **60 Minutes** fame is coming into your facility, with cameras and crew. He's coming down the hall with all of his equipment, and it's suddenly crystal clear that he's coming to *your* department. Since your department is food service, you rationalize that perhaps he's hungry. He's not. He says, "We hear your food service department is terrible," and then shoves the microphone in your face. Do you want to respond to Mike, and his millions of viewers, with a puny "We do a great job. Everyone is very happy." Of course not. You want to be able to quickly provide solid data that prove, beyond a shadow of a doubt, that not only do you serve a good product, but the service is excellent as well:

- Of patients, 85% ranked the food above average or excellent.

- Of patients, 87% expressed satisfaction with the menu, service, and presentation style.

- A PI team measured the time it takes to go through the cafeteria line, and, for those people who could decide what they wanted to eat, they were able to complete their transaction in an average of 3.5 minutes, 1.5 minutes less than the "acceptable target" set by customers.

- All patients at nutritional risk were assessed by a dietitian and received appropriate nutrition.

- Inpatient meals were delivered as scheduled ($\pm$3 minutes) 97% of the time.

Of course, there are other reasons, besides Mike Wallace, to measure and have solid data available. For one, more and more managers are seeing the value of using data (rather than funny-inside-feelings) to drive their management decisions and performance improvement efforts. Two, managed care companies and businesses that purchase managed care plans will be focusing their attention on two key pieces of data: (1) outcomes and (2) cost performance. They want to know which provider is producing the best clinical outcomes and, among the best producers, who has the lowest cost.

Data-Driven Management

We need to know:

- *How we're performing and why we're there*

- *How our performance compares to others*

- *Where we want to be*

- *Which process has the best track record and is most likely to get us where we want to go*

- *If desired results were achieved*

In an immature managed care market—a situation most states are currently experiencing—reducing cost is the first priority. One reason, of course, is economics. A second, less obvious, reason is simply because cost data are available, while clinical outcome data are temporarily scarce.

Scarce data, combined with increasing demand for it, has made clinical outcome data a hot commodity. Experts say it will be years before nationally-linked databases are able to provide reliable, usable, severity-adjusted data. In the absence of ideal data, however, organizations (e.g., managed care organizations (MCOs), businesses, newspapers) will, out of necessity, use whatever is available to rate and rank providers' care. This necessity is igniting the birth of a cottage industry devoted exclusively to data. In states with Sunshine acts, all discharge data, which include diagnosis, length of stay (LOS), charges, mortality, etc., are public information. Data entrepreneurs can access or buy it and then turn around and sell it to businesses, MCOs, TV stations, and others. Some sell it in its raw form, and others analyze it first.

The example in Figure 3.1 shows how physicians' performance can be analyzed and compared to one another. Adjusted for severity, it displays comparative cost and length of stay data and shows, what many have suspected, that reduced LOS does not necessarily guarantee lower costs. On the other hand, physicians who were able to keep costs down, regardless of LOS (gray area), were regarded positively. The addition of successful outcome performance data to this equation makes the provider even more attractive to purchasers of healthcare services—high-quality outcomes within acceptable cost limits—the goal all customers can buy into from the patient receiving care to the MCO that pays the bills.

Thus, healthcare providers need to be proactive, not only in designing systems that reliably deliver high-quality care at the lowest possible cost but

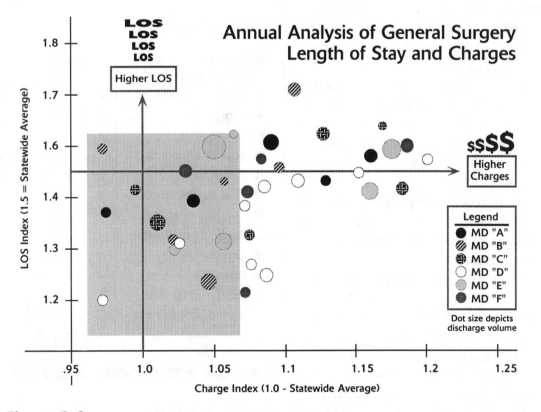

Figure 3.1
Annual Analysis of General Surgery Length of Stay (LOS) and Charges

also in verifying and documenting the extent of their success so they can benchmark, compare themselves with competitors, review and analyze providers with excessive LOS, and market to all types of potential customers.

Data Collection, Display, and Analysis

This chapter, **Measurement**, and the next chapter, **Assessment**, both deal with and rely heavily on data collection, display, and analysis. As a prelude to these sections, we'll review some basics by answering some frequently asked questions (FAQs).

What are data collection, display, and analysis?

A way to back up and document assumptions and perceptions about performance results with actual information or data.

For what purpose are data collection, display, and analysis used?

- Comparing actual outcome and process results to preset targets
- Targeting potential improvement opportunities
- Determining if a team is needed
- Illustrating what is happening

When should data collection, display, and analysis be used?

- Routine assessment of performance results
- As needed, to help analyze unstable outcomes or processes
- Recurring or common cause problems and cross-functional processes

There are many methods for data collection, display, and analysis. How do I know which one to use?

First, decide what data or information you need—the data that will verify, or possibly negate, an assumption. Then look over the list of **Data Tools**, Exhibit 3.1. After you use them for a while, you will get a feel for which one to use when, but until then, use the one you like and understand how to

Data tools

Can be used to:	Collect	Display	Analyze
■ Surveys (written, phone, interview)	x		x
■ Fishbone diagram	x		
■ Sampling	x		
■ Observation	x		
■ Task or checklists	x		
■ Checksheets	x	x	x
■ Cost-benefit analysis	x	x	x
■ Run (a.k.a. trend)		x	x
■ Pie and bar charts		x	x
■ Control charts		x	x
■ Histograms	x	x	x
■ Scatter diagrams	x	x	x
■ Pareto diagrams		x	x
■ Flowcharts	x	x	x

Exhibit 3.1 Methods for Data Collection, Display, and Analysis

use properly. Information and blank copies of the tools listed will be given within the text of the book or in **Appendix A.**

Data collection seems laborious. Is there any way to avoid it?

Yes, too frequently, data are tediously collected when they already exist somewhere else in the organization. Always check first to see if they're available—and assessable. Be sure, however, if you use someone else's data, that they are reliable, timely enough, and relevant. Also, as a courtesy, let the party who is sharing his or her data with you know why you are collecting the data and what will be done with the information. Also, offer to share any new information when the project is complete.

How can the data collection task be shared by team members?

Standardized and piloted forms facilitate sharing data collection among several people. As long as they've been tested for *reliability* and *validity,* the integrity of the effort will be maintained.

How can we test the reliability and validity of our data collection?

Conduct a pilot study using the standardized form. After, ask the following:
- Was the form found to be understandable and efficient by users?
- Was the form *reliable* (i.e., when several people measured the same indicator, collecting from the same source, did they come up with the same answer)?
- Was the form *valid* (i.e., Were measurements useful and meaningful to the user? Did measures remain constant? Were data results used? Did feedback lead to improvements in performance results?

These answers may not come quickly. Testing, trial and error, and use over time determine validity and reliability, not just expert opinion.

How do I know if the sample size is adequate?

In 1994 the Joint Commission provided a guideline, "If the average number of cases per quarter is more than 600, at least 5% of cases are reviewed; and if the average number of cases per quarter is fewer than 600, at least 30 cases are reviewed."[1] But it is often situational. Some believe that you should collect as much data as you need to collect to convince whomever you need to convince. This may be more or less than the Joint Commission suggests. Play it safe. Check with the data gurus at your organization, and see if a guideline exists. The goal is to have enough data to learn from and make a point, but not too much. No one wants to give up their day job to collect data. Nor does anyone want to wade through an unnecessary amount of data.

What should be measured?

The answer to this question is the same answer you would want to give to Mike Wallace if he came to visit. Measure key performance results—display *evidence* that the department, unit, critical path team, pain treatment team, and so forth were able to meet or exceed all of the outcomes selected by the clinical staff and the customer, followed the recommended process, and were able to do so while staying within their cost and resource limitations.

The outcome, process, and cost *indicators* that were created back in Chapter 1 of the book, as guides, are now useful again, in another capacity: measures. For each outcome, process, or cost indicator, the question can be posed: Was it met, not met, or exceeded? In other words, if you say your outcomes, processes, and costs are terrific, you should be able to prove it *with evidence*. Thus, the answer to the question, "What should I measure?" is an easy one if you've taken the time to identify outcome, process, and cost indicators.

Remember, the factor that distinguishes an indicator from a desire is the ability to measure objectively (with support of evidence) whether or not the goal has been met or exceeded. The goal may be a desired clinical outcome, a preferred process to follow, or a cost target. Referencing the outcome indicator in Exhibit 3.2 a patient is either able to verbalize knowledge of exercise, pulse, and take-home medications, or not. It also won't matter if the evaluator *feels* negative or biased about the situation, because the patient either has the knowledge, or does not. The clinical outcome was met, or not.

Care or Service **Outcome Indicators**	Performance or **Process Indicators**	**Financial Indicators**
Care (clinical and satisfaction) or service results	Recommended process and employee responsibilities	Necessary or avoidable cost

Strategic Priority: Become the cardiovascular care provider of choice in the community.
Performance Improvement Priority: Reduce patient readmissions by increasing their knowledge of their disease.

Knowledge standard: *Each patient will receive information related to his/her condition and care of that condition.*	**Evaluation standard:** *Each nurse will evaluate patient's response and outcomes.*	**Resource standard:** *Resources will be available and utilized appropriately.*
Discharge knowledge indicator: *Each patient will be able to verbalize, prior to discharge, knowledge of exercise, pulse, and take home medications.*	**Implementation/evaluation indicator:** *Each nurse will document discharge knowledge status in the patient's record upon discharge.*	**Resource indicator:** *Flexible budget targets met ± 2% for paid direct hours or Productivity indicator: 30 minutes (on the average)*

Exhibit 3.2 Indicator Development Worksheet Example

*The words, "**as evidenced by...?**" are*
an invaluable addition to every manager's vocabulary.

Typically, managers measure outcomes—almost always *clinical outcomes* and, somewhat less enthusiastically, *cost outcomes*. It's a good place to start, but its not the whole answer. There are two reasons. One, when the *outcome* is not met, it usually (some experts say 85% of the time) has something to do with the *process*. Two, when the *outcome* is met there is a tendency to assume that the *process* is working and that everyone followed it. While this is generally true, gurus of performance improvement insist that even good processes can be improved. It is important to measure the *process* as well as the outcome. Are people following the process? Is the process delivering the desired level of performance that is needed and wanted?

What data should be collected?

The answer to this question is not as straightforward as one would think. Once a decision is made about what should be measured, figuring out what data to collect should be very clear; sometimes it is. Recall for a moment the example in Exhibit 3.2 of the patient being able to verbalize knowledge of exercise, pulse, and take-home medications. What actual data should be collected? Should patients be given a written test so their scores can be reviewed? Should the nurse check in with the home health caregiver to find out if the patient has made errors in self-administering medications? Should the readmits due to medication error be counted? Which data will be the best indicator of whether or not the desired outcome was achieved?

Obviously, it's an important question. Few of us have extra time on our hands to collect unnecessary data. If data have to be collected (and they do), we want to spend as little time doing it as possible. Thus, it's important to zero in on the right data, the data that will give the best picture of what is really going on for that particular population of patients. Many times, data are collected because they are easiest, or they are the most available, or they are mistakenly thought to be required. That's why the Mike Wallace analogy works. It forces a defense and a reach for the most significant information available.

While common sense and familiarity with desired outcomes is always a good place to start, there are other tools available as well. Comparative clinical data indicator projects, fishbone diagrams, and task lists also help identify and prioritize potential data so the most promising data can be collected first.

Using External Sources for Data: Comparative Data and Information

One way to figure out what data to collect is by referencing a comparative performance data initiative. There are many comparative data indicator projects in existence today. The oldest (1985), and largest, with over 1000 members, is the Quality Indicator (QI) Project®, operated by the Maryland Hospital Association. Their initial mission was to "explore and develop valid and reliable ways to monitor care, conduct comparative analysis, and identify opportunities for improvement." As shown in Exhibit 3.3, the project currently supplies members with 15 outcomes-based clinical performance indicators (10 inpatient, 5 ambulatory) and 7 psychiatric care indicators for evaluation. Additional sets of indicators are in various stages of development.

Participating organizations report data results quarterly, and in return, the Project staff compiles aggregate data and other feedback for industrywide comparisons. Feedback is provided via quarterly reports that are used to compare aggregate rates, as well as longitudinal trending. If an organization wants to compare itself with a more narrowly defined peer group, custom reports can be created. The QI Project® also provides participants with training and user-friendly software to help ease data collection and submission.[2]

The need for a unified, reliable national database is evident. Taking the lead, the Joint Commission embarked a decade ago on the Agenda for Change, "an initiative that eventually led to the creation of the Indicator Measurement System (IMSystem) whose collection of tested indicators is focused primarily on acute care settings." In its January 23, 1996, news release, the Joint Commission announced its "intent to include a group of acceptable measurement systems in its accreditation process under a single performance measurement umbrella. An important objective of this plan will be to preserve the element of choice for the accredited organization by allowing it to select the approved measurement system that best meets its needs."[3]

In support of this initiative, the Joint Commission has created a National Library of Healthcare Indicators (NLHI), "a comprehensive indicator catalog that includes performance measures judged by content experts to have face validity for application to various types of healthcare organizations." The March 5, 1996, news release continues by quoting Dennis S. O'Leary, M.D., president, Joint Commission , "The development of NLHI extends the Joint Commission's decade-long commitment to implementing an outcomes-oriented accreditation process that provides a continuing stimulus to quality

The Quality Indicator Project®

Quality Indicator Project® Indicators

Inpatient Indicators

I Hospital Acquired Infections

II Surgical Site Infections

III Inpatient Mortality

IV Neonatal Mortality

V Perioperative Mortality

VI Cesarean Sections

VII Unscheduled Readmissions within 31 Days for the Same or Related Condition

VIII Unscheduled Admissions Following Ambulatory Procedure

IX Unscheduled Returns to a Special Care Unit during the Same Inpatient Admission

X Unscheduled Returns to Operating Room during the Same Inpatient Admission

Ambulatory Indicators

A-1 Unscheduled Returns to the Emergency Department (ED) Within 72 Hours for the Same or Related Condition

A-2 Registered Patients in the ED Greater than Six Hours

A-3 ED Cases Where Discrepancy between Initial and Final X-Ray Reports Required an Adjustment in Patient Management

A-4 Registered Patients Who Leave the ED Prior to Completion of Treatment

A-5 Cancellation of Ambulatory Procedure on the Day of the Procedure

Psychiatric Care Indicators

PSY-I Injurious Behaviors (Adult Units)

PSY-II Unplanned Departures (Adult)

PSY-III Transfers to Acute Care Unit (Adult)

PSY-IV Readmissions within 15 days (Adult)

PSY-V Injurious Behaviors (Adolescent Units)

PSY-VI Unplanned Departures (Adolescent)

PSY-VII Readmissions within 15 days (Adolescent)

Current Research Initiatives

Long-Term Care Indicators

LTC-I Unplanned Weight Change

LTC-III Skin Integrity

LTC-III Documented Unassisted Falls

LTC-IV Unplanned Transfers to Acute Care Setting

LTC-V Infection Incidence

LTC-VI Changes in Mobility

Exhibit 3.3 Quality Improvement Project® of the Maryland Hospital Association
Information supplied by the Quality Indicator Project.® Used with permission.

improvement."[4] This concept is discussed in more detail in Exhibit 3.4., **Joint Commission: National Library of Healthcare Indicators**.

After individual performance measurement systems (PMSs)—such as the QI Project®)—meet Joint Commission evaluation criteria and are approved, individual organizations can select an approved PMS and whatever applicable indicators within that system that match their needs. Organizations can use any PMS as long as it has met the Joint Commission criteria.

Healthcare organizations benefit from using external databases for comparative purposes in several ways. One, performance assessment conducted solely on an internal basis is likely to give a distorted view of performance. A facility might think it's doing well because of continual improvements in a particular area. External comparisons, however, might reveal that the facility actually lags far behind its peers for that same area. Trending and comparing clinical performance data among hundreds of similar acute-care hospitals give new insight to internal quality improvement efforts. Two, managed care companies, as they mature, are looking at more than just money. Their goal is to find the best care at the lowest cost. Indicator projects afford hospitals an opportunity to compare themselves to other similar organizations, to assess how well they're doing. Three, the Joint Commission's information management standards (IM.10) also require participation in "external reference databases for comparative purposes."[5]

Comparative performance data projects help organizations by suggesting what data are important to collect; showing variances in performance from expected patterns, from the norm, and from the best of the best; and detecting, through data analysis, an organization's strengths, vision, and future potential. Last, the direction of the Joint Commission is clear. The accreditation process will become increasingly outcomes-oriented. The outcomes will become public record. Finally, businesses, MCOs, and the public at large will be able be make data-based, data-driven decisions.

So what's the problem? The biggest challenge facing comparative performance data projects, or *performance measurement systems* as they are also called, is figuring out how to level the playing field, to ensure apples are being compared to apples and oranges to oranges. Adjusting for severity and testing for reliability are complex challenges. Fortunately, there are experts at the Joint Commission and the performance measurement systems—like the QI Project®—who relish taking on this challenge. Those of us who burned our statistics textbook while proclaiming, "This has nothing to do with real life," will forever be in their debt.

Joint Commission
National Library of Healthcare Indicators

In a promising step forward, the Joint Commission on Accreditation of Healthcare Organizations (Joint Commission) is in the process of creating a National Library of Healthcare Indicators (NLHI). Pioneering an unprecedented collaborative effort, they have solicited indicators for inclusion from provider organizations*, professional associations, educational institutions, purchasers, database developers, government agencies, health service researchers, and others. In their own words:

> NLHI is a comprehensive indicator catalogue which presents standardized profiles of performance measures judged by content experts to have face validity for application to various types of healthcare organizations.
> Over time, the Library is expected to serve as a continuous source of promising measures for evaluating performance in health care. Initial users are expected to be purchasers and health care organizations themselves. Later, the indicators most appropriate for accreditation purposes will be made available to performance measurement systems approved for inclusion in the Joint Commission's accreditation process.

Dennis S. O'Leary, M.D., president, Joint Commission, characterizes the Library as a continuous supply source of indicators for the Joint Commission's IMSystem and other performance measurement systems endorsed by their Council on Performance Measurement. "This will substantially enhance our abilities to support quality improvement in health care organizations while also setting the stage for using performance measures in the accreditation process."

Indicator performance categories
- **Administrative/Financial**
  Performance measures that address the coordination and integration of functions, services and activities across operational components
- **Clinical Performance**
  Performance measures that address the care processes and outcomes for specific conditions and procedures
- **Health Status**
  Performance measures that address the functional well-being of specific populations, both in general and in relation to specific conditions
- **Satisfaction**
  Performance measures that address how well patient/enrollee, purchaser and practitioner needs are met

Indicator Integration Into the Future Accreditation Process

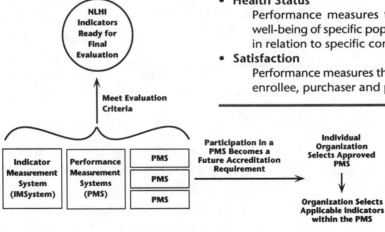

* Providers include acute care, ambulatory care, behavioral healthcare, home care, and long-term care.

Exhibit 3.4 Joint Commission National Library of Healthcare Indicators (NLHI)
Information extracted from a Joint Commission News Release, April 17, 1996: 1–2. Used with permission.

Fishbone Diagrams

A second way to identify data for collection is a method called *Ishikawa's cause-and-effect diagram*, more popularly known as the *fishbone diagram*. Fishbone diagrams are used primarily to brainstorm "possible" root causes (see Figure 3.2) of a recurring problem or to identify and clarify problems. In both cases, the outcome is more information on what data to collect. The goal in creating a fishbone is to get increasingly more specific; the "why technique" is used to press deeper and deeper into sub-issues. After the ideas are brainstormed, the group can use multivoting or another technique to prioritize the ideas and help the team reach consensus on the potential cause.

Once prioritized by the team, data can be collected to confirm or refute their perception. It is not uncommon for a perception to prove false, even when the group is 100% confident that "X" is the cause or at the root of the issue. This is particularly true with recurring problems. A cause is assumed, and the solution is applied—with no improvement—because it's the wrong cause. It would be like trying to fix a broken arm by putting the cast on a hand. Many managers "rush to solution" by assuming a root cause and quickly apply a solution because they've been influenced, over the years, to come up with quick fixes. However, when one adds up all the time spent fixing and refixing the same problem over and over—not to mention the avoidable cost of quality—it's easy to see the cost-effectiveness of assigning a team of subject matter experts to the task of solving the problem forever.

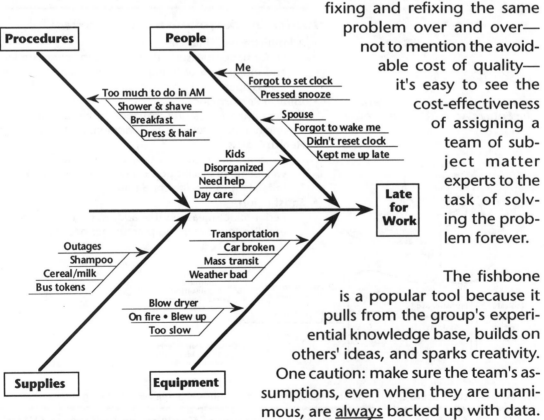

The fishbone is a popular tool because it pulls from the group's experiential knowledge base, builds on others' ideas, and sparks creativity. One caution: make sure the team's assumptions, even when they are unanimous, are <u>always</u> backed up with data.

Figure 3.2 Fishbone Example

Task Lists

A task list is a simple action plan. Most people use task lists (a.k.a., checklists), in their day-to-day routine—grocery lists, do today, skills checklists, for example. In process analysis, it helps team members organize their data collection. It is most often used to generate a list of data (to collect) that will help analyze and confirm the root cause of a problem, but it can also be used to generate a list of problems or processes to improve, possible solutions, and indicators to monitor.

The task list in Exhibit 3.5 is from a team working on improving customer service and waiting times in the emergency department (ED). The initial assumption was that the waiting time was solely the fault of the ED. After deeper investigation, the team realized it was a patient flow problem—patients were backing up in the ED waiting for beds in the ICU. The ICU group said they had patients waiting to transfer to the floors, but beds were routinely not available. Why? Patients on the floors were being discharged early enough, according to their charts, but at 5:00 PM they were still there. The team, after prioritizing the fishbone, flowchart, and some other work, used consensus to select the most probable root causes. Then they listed the (collectable) data that would confirm or deny their suspicions, and for each assumption, they selected data.

Before they collected the data, however, they asked if the data were already available or collected by some other source. If the source is reliable, it's far better to borrow data than to duplicate the effort and waste time. If data need to be collected, what method will be used? How will data be collected? It's an important question and there are four different approaches that can be taken: (1) sampling, (2) survey, (3) observation, and (4) checksheets. They will be looked at individually in the next section. Last, once the "what" and "how" questions are answered, target dates for completion and names of the people who are responsible for the results can be added to complete the action plan.

1. What data do we need to analyze?	2. Where is it? Will we borrow data or collect?	3. How will data be collected? Survey, Observation Sampling, Checksheet?
Problem: Late discharges are slowing the patient flow and backing up patients in ICU and the ED		
Late discharges per day	On nursing units Collect	Observation and checksheet
Why patients remain in room postdischarge	Patients can provide this info. Collect	Survey: written, interview, or both
What would motivate them to go home?	Patients, MDs nursing staff Collect	Survey: written, oral, or both
Is it occurring on all nursing units?	In the task force records Borrow	NA

Exhibit 3.5 Task List Example

Processes for Collecting Data

Four of the easiest and most popular ways to collect data are (1) sampling, (2) survey, (3) observation, and (4) checksheets. There are other methods, but for the majority of us who have statisticphobia, this is a good place to start. If an issue is that big, that technical, that important to require sophisticated statistical analysis, then it's important enough to seek assistance from experts for that project. For our purposes, we'll focus on these methods because they are easy, time efficient, and useful.

Something about sampling. Sampling, by definition, is a piece or item that is able to show the quality of the whole. After eating a bite of a sandwich, one generally knows if he or she wants to eat more, based on that "sample." Sampling is probably the most often used method of collecting data. It is popular because it streamlines a laborious process. The simplest way to understand sampling is with a bag of M&Ms. *Random* sampling is when one reaches into the bag (blindfolded) and grabs one piece of candy. To *stratify* the sample, we might pull out all but the brown candies and then reach in blindfolded to randomly select a piece from the remaining brown candy. An example of *systematic* sampling would be to take every third or fourth piece of candy. Types of sampling can be used alone or in combination. For example, a sample might be stratified by age (21–30 years) and then further narrowed by random or systematic selection. Or every 10th person might be taken from the phone book (systematic) and then called if their name begins with a vowel. The goal is to narrow the field to a sample small enough to study but large enough to be valid, as we discussed at the beginning of this chapter. Exhibit 3.6 has some more examples and information about sampling.

Surveys. Is there anyone out there who hasn't been surveyed ad nauseam? Daily, it seems, we get bombarded with phone surveys, postcards, letters, and people stopping us in shopping malls. Even television programs ask us to phone in our opinions… for a charge. Everyone is looking for answers, information, something that will help them make better business decisions. Even though it can be aggravating, most of us are seduced by the belief that some improvement will be made if we contribute our war stories, information, or suggestions. However, have any of you ever received feedback from a survey that you participated in, telling the outcomes and what would be changed as a result of the new information? It happens a lot less often than the survey, but when it does, we feel gratified because we've effected a change for the positive. Keep that thought in mind as you prepare surveys and ask people to take the time to complete them. Some other important survey suggestions follow:

Sampling

Random Sampling

A portion of data is selected by chance from the entire database, and each item has an equal chance of being selected. **Example**: *Pulling a name out of a fishbowl that holds 100% of employee names.*

Stratified Sampling

Data are divided into groups—an age or geographical group, a diagnosis-related group (DRG), or a physician group (all surgeons)—and then each group is sampled separately using a random or systematic technique. **Example**: *Pulling randomly (or systematically) out of a fishbowl that holds only male employee names.*

Systematic Sampling

Every X^{th} item or every Y^{th} time period is sampled. This seems easy, but if the total sample is not sorted randomly, it will lead to inaccurate or skewed data. **Example**: *Pulling names out of a fishbowl that holds 100% of employee names, but only using every 5th name.*

Nonprobability Sampling

Subject matter experts make a qualitative judgment and assumptions about a common issue in order to reduce the size of the sample, assuming that the problem is uniform:
- *Convenience sampling: e.g., all patients admitted last week*
- *Purposive sampling: e.g., all patients over 20 who have measles*
- *Quota sampling: e.g., 5% of female breast cancer patients 55–65*

Generally

1. *The sample must be large enough to reliably answer questions about the population and satisfy those who will be scrutinizing.*

2. *The smaller the sample, the less accurate it is likely to be.*

3. *When it's necessary to be very accurate, consult with experts who work in your organization. They can be excellent resources to your team.*

4. *For efficiency, samples should be small without losing needed representation. Generally, at least 30 cases or 5% of the population, whichever is greater.[6]*

Exhibit 3.6 Sampling Overview

Survey Suggestions

- *Keep it short; focus in on what is really important and show respect for others' time.*

- *Use a standardized format. This is especially important with verbal surveys.*

- *Test the survey ahead of time for bias and validity.*

- *Use an acceptable survey size.*

- *Offer to share results, and then do it.*

- *Make sure there's something to be gained for the customer.*

- *Do something with the information, and then communicate it to the survey participants.*

Exhibits 3.7 through 3.9 and Figure 3.3 are part of a survey sent to a group of coninuous quality improvement (CQI) customers. Out of respect for the customers' time, the survey was kept to one page, and survey respondents were asked if they would like to receive results. While some surveyors send a dollar or a pen to entice participation, M&Ms were sent with this survey. And it worked! Sixty percent of the surveys were returned. It was a simple matter of knowing customers and what would motivate them to take time out of their busy day to fill out a survey. The feedback was extraordinary—it was obvious that people took time and really thought about their responses (even though none of us knew they would one day be published). Exhibits 3.8, 3.9, and Figure 3.3 show the results that were gleaned from the survey and, as promised, results were shared with participants. In addition to being an example of a survey and results, there is some useful information about implementing CQI from some very smart customers.

Probably the most important surveys managers do are customer feedback surveys, which include everything from whether the patient was happy to whether the clinical outcomes were met. Most managers are familiar with the process of surveying their *external* customers. Patient satisfaction surveys, indicator performance measures, physician report cards, and the like are all examples of customer feedback surveys that are frequently used by healthcare organizations. It is not unusual for patients to be bombarded with surveys, phone calls, and requests for suggestions, so a coordinated, integrated system would, no doubt, increase participation. There are several

Survey

Healthcare organizations have been actively implementing performance improvement systems for several years, long enough to assess what is working and what's not. For organizations that are "up and running," the task of sustaining organizational momentum — the topic of this survey — continues to be an ongoing challenge.

1. How successful has your organization been in sustaining CQI momentum – in terms of values <u>and</u> measurable results?

1	2	3	4	5	6	7	8	9	10
What's CQI?									**Very Successful**

2. Looking at the list below, put an "**S**" next to the strategies or factors that you feel contributed to your **success** and a "**D**" next to those you would approach **differently** if you had it to do again.

        a. Identifying and developing indicators of outcome, process, and cost   _____

        b. Leadership commitment and support   _____

        c. Mid-level management team leader tools and group process training   _____

        d. Ongoing mid-level management involvement   _____

        e. In-house facilitator training for ongoing support   _____

        f. Culture development   _____

        g. Communication planning and follow-up   _____

        h. Organizing and communicating measurement systems   _____

        i. Planning for and pacing change   _____

        j. Ongoing education, practice support, and coaching   _____

        k. Other _____ _____

        l. Other _____ _____

3. **What was the most important lesson you learned?**

4. Many believers in TQM/CQI contend that if you do the right thing the right way the first time, increased efficiency and profitability can occur concurrently. To what extent have you found this to be true?

1	2	3	4	5	6	7	8	9	10
We improved performance but it was costly (time/money)							**We made enormous gains in performance and productivity**		

5. Managers in our organization have successfully used CQI (and/or other performance improvement methods) to:
    Check all that apply: ❑ Meet JCAHO standards ❑ Improve quality/performance outcomes ❑ Reduce costs

_____

Check one: CIO or COO ____ Vice Pres. ____ Quality Coordinator ____ Mid-level Manager ____

Hospital: Under 100 beds ____ Over 100 beds ____ Home Care Agency ____ Other _____

Please send me: ❑ Survey results   ❑ Current workshop & consulting info (propaganda)

_____ _____ _____
Name   Title   Organization

_____ _____
Address   City/State/Zip

          ❧ **Return in this handy mailer or fax to (305) 383-0034... by June 15th please** ❧

Exhibit 3.7 Customer Feedback Survey

Results

I now have valid statistical evidence that **M&M's**, combined with **guilt**, works! 60% of the surveys were returned... an incredible response for which I am most grateful. I particularly appreciated the personal notes and anecdotes... of both struggles and celebrations. For those of you who aren't getting the results you want, now may be the time to take me up on my free telephone consults as I am off the road until the end of August. Last, if you are receiving this, it is because you checked the box marked "send survey results," so I'll now prep you for the *data*. 34 surveys arrived early enough to include in the tabulation. The responses in questions 1, 2, and 4 add up to 34. The responses in #5 do not because 0-3 answers could be selected. One survey lacked demographic info, thus only 33 responses for #s 6, 7. The raw data is below. Lessons learned and analysis follow.

1. How successful has your organization been in sustaining CQI momentum – in terms of values <u>and</u> measurable results?

N=34

1 What's CQI?	2	3	4	5	6	7	8	9	10 Very Successful
	2	1	2	5	2	9	10		3

2. **Legend**: S= strategies or factors that contributed to **success**. D = things you'd approach differently. NA = no answer. I = still working on this. D† = more of it. D* = employee component. D** = changed CEO mid-process. **Order has been changed to highlight contributors to success.**

	S	D	NA	I	D†	D*	D**
b. Leadership commitment and support	24	9	-	-	-	-	1
c. Mid-level management team leader tools and group process training	22	11	-	-	-	1	-
d. Ongoing mid-level management involvement	21	11	1	-	1	-	-
f. Culture development	19	15	-	-	-	-	-
a. Identifying and developing indicators of outcome, process, and cost	18	13	1	1	1	-	-
j. Ongoing education, practice support, and coaching	17	14	2	-	1	-	-
g. Communication planning and follow-up	15	17	-	-	1	1	-
e. In-house facilitator training for ongoing support	15	18	-	-	1	-	-
h. Organizing and communicating measurement systems	13	19	1	1	-	-	-
i. Planning for and pacing change	12	21	1	-	-	-	-
k. Other: Results tracking and reporting	1	-	-	-	-	-	-
m. Other: Did not buy into a particular Guru to follow	1	-	-	-	-	-	-
l. Other: Physician involvement	-	1	-	-	-	-	-

3. What was the most important lesson you learned? *See reverse side.*

4. Many believers in TQM/CQI contend that if you do the right thing the right way the first time, increased efficiency and profitability can occur concurrently. To what extent have you found this to be true?

N=34

1	2	3	4	5	6	7	8	9	10	NA
		1		2	3	11	10	3		4

We improved performance but it was costly (time/money) — We made enormous gains in performance and productivity

5. Managers in our organization have successfully used CQI (and/or other performance improvement methods) to: Check all that apply: ☐ Meet JCAHO standards ☐ Improve quality/performance outcomes ☐ Reduce costs

30 88%   30 88%   20 59%

6. Check one: CEO or COO _3_ Vice Pres. _13_ Quality Coordinator _10_ Mid-level Manager _7_

7. Hospital: Under 100 beds _3_ Over 100 beds _29_ Home Care Agency __ Other _1_

❧ **P.S. If you requested propaganda, but did not receive it, call (305) 382-1283. It's because I didn't have your name/address.** ❧

Exhibit 3.8 Customer Feedback Survey Results

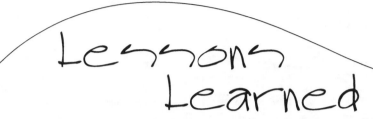

Comments on leadership...

We must have leadership commitment and resources devoted • Leadership is crucial for making the CQI process work • Must, must, must have top down involvement... not just support • Can't move fast enough. Only use "stretch" goals. Less does not inspire • There needs to be a highly structured organizational plan, i.e. prioritizing teams and results accountability • ...that commitment, support, and involvement is necessary top down and bottom up; that some things are inappropriately put into CQI process; that process is important! • Leadership commitment is essential. Also you must plan, plan, plan! • Consistency of, and commitment to approach used and <u>constant</u> effort to development and group improvement efforts • The most important factor in success is support of the facility leadership • Middle managers are the most resistant group and need to be involved early in planning stages • Need more time spent in planning • You can never start CQI implementation too soon • The importance of mid-level manager buy in. Without it you cannot get line staff free to participate in teams nor will corrective action plans be sanctioned and supported.

Comments on communication...

Communicate TQM/CQI philosophy and use tools as a means to the end. Insure that executive management "walks the talk" and uses tools and methods routinely, so they're part of the organization's culture • Focus must be on the benefits the CQI process brings for staff to engage in it • Never under estimate the importance of staff participation and communication • Communication is so important. Need to verify a common language • Go slow with staff and do CQI with staff people <u>before</u> you tell them they are already doing it (CQI scares people, but the process is easy!).

Comments on cross-functional teams...

Understanding and gaining the perspective of other disciplines is essential in effecting support and cooperation on achieving a positive outcome • The importance of the team approach with all levels of employees working toward a common goal • It takes a lot of time and effort to get people to sustain the CQI process • Keep at it (follow up)! • I <u>love</u> seeing employees taking such an ownership in their teams! CQI really works and employees appreciate being able to participate! • Not to try and solve world problems with initial CQI teams • The tools • The investment of employees in performance improvement is <u>critical</u> to success • Empowering staff not only helps us make the right decisions, but improves the morale of the staff.

Comments on education and training ...

The education must be on-going for all staff. Turnover hurts the process. The addition of a third facility was also difficult with new CEO and manager changes • Timing of training is central to its success. CQI/TQM is as much attitude as techniques. Organizations need to shape TQM to fit them rather than feel as though they have to "do it by the book." • Would have provided more training on coping with change • Need more time spent on education.

Miscellaneous comments ...

- Roll with the punches. We didn't do the right things the right way the first time. We're back on track now.
- We could not get the institution to move after our very exciting education sessions. Administration pulled back all the way.
- Healthcare is dynamic just like change and what you think you know today is totally new tomorrow.
- The process and techniques really do work, but must be applied consistently all the time.
- Need to develop indicators of outcome, process, and cost and hold leaders accountable.
- The "stuff" that is meaningful or worthwhile or useful sticks – the rest disappears.
- The overall investment (time/dollars) should have been better researched.
- We need lots more work. We now are at the beginning phase of integration with another facility. Stress, anxiety are extreme.
- Measure baseline elements.

Exhibit 3.9 Customer Feedback Survey Results: Lessons Learned

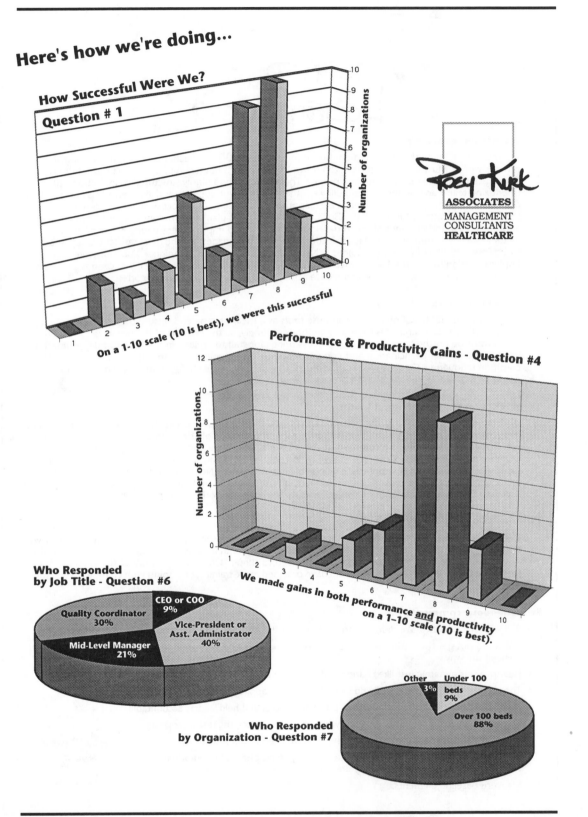

Figure 3.3 Customer Feedback Survey Results: Graphics

key external customers (patients, visitors, physicians, third-party payers, etc.) and the more healthcare organizations know about their level of satisfaction, the easier it will be to build systems and make improvements in pursuit of their satisfaction.

However, external customers aren't the only customers. Meeting the needs and expectations of *internal* customers (other departments, functions, our employees, our managers) is as important as meeting the expectations of external customers. In fact, in many cases, if the internal customers' needs aren't met, they, in turn, become incapable of meeting their external customers' needs (i.e., an undelivered supply item may prevent a care giver from performing an ordered task on a patient).

Exhibits 3.10, 3.11, and 3.12 are all *internal* customer feedback forms. The **Internal Customer Survey**, Exhibit 3.10, is used to assess the performance of other departments or functions. Some functions are invisible to external customers. People who work in human resources, maintenance, and pharmacy, for example, may never actually come in contact with patients, visitors, physicians, or payers. Yet their impact on outcomes can be as important as that of the direct caregiver, their internal customer. An incorrect medication dose sent to a patient-care unit is an example with a potentially huge avoidable cost of quality. If the nursing staff catches the error, the cost of repairing it is frustrating but small. However, if it's not caught, it can cost the patient anxiety, discomfort, and who knows what else. It can cost the nurse, pharmacist, physician, and coordinator time to resolve the issue and follow up. (This is one of many examples that demonstrate that doing something right the first time is not just nice for the customers; it's nice for providers and the bottom line.) Because of this, many organizations are now asking their front-line staff (who actually connect with customers) to evaluate other departments, functions, and individuals who support (or fail to support) them in their work, using the customer-driven indicators developed in Chapter 1.

The **Feedback for Senior Management** and **Feedback for Senior Management Results** (Exhibits 3.11 and 3.12) are used by managers to assess the performance of senior management, and in turn, is used by staff members to assess their manager's performance. The 360° assessment, as it is sometimes called, is a growing trend among organizations that place a high value on the internal customer-supplier relationship and its impact on organizational outcomes. Remember, just as in relay races, the handoff from one function to the other has a powerful impact on overall outcomes, and that handoff may be from one function to another function or from manager to employee.

Internal Customer Survey

My department's key customers	What they expect from us
_____	_____
_____	_____
_____	_____

	NEVER				ALWAYS
1. I know who my internal customers are and what we need to do to meet or exceed their expectations.	1	2	3	4	5
2. Decisions are made in light of the identified needs of our:					
Key external customers (patients, physicians, third-party payers)	1	2	3	4	5
Key internal customers (other departments and functions)	1	2	3	4	5
3. We meet the needs of internal and external customers in a balanced manner.	1	2	3	4	5
4. We ask internal customers what they need and want on a regular basis...	1	2	3	4	5
5. ... and we listen, sincerely, to understand their needs.	1	2	3	4	5
6. We respond to internal customer requests and identified needs routinely meeting predetermined expectations.	1	2	3	4	5
7. We exceed expectations by anticipating and responding to internal customer needs before they are verbalized.	1	2	3	4	5

My department's key suppliers	What I can expect from them
1. _____	_____
2. _____	_____
3. _____	_____

1. I know who my internal suppliers are.	1	2	3	4	5
2. I know what I can expect from them.	1	2	3	4	5
3. They meet or exceed my expectations.	1	2	3	4	5

Exhibit 3.10 Internal Customer Survey   *(Continues)*

The following questions will help you assess the performance of your individual suppliers.

Supplier number 1...

NEVER   ALWAYS

1. Makes decisions in light of our department's stated needs.   1   2   3   4   5

2. Asks our department what we need or want on a regular basis... 1   2   3   4   5

3. ... and they listen, sincerely, to understand our needs.   1   2   3   4   5

4. Responds to our department's requests and identified needs   1   2   3   4   5
   routinely meeting our predetermined expectations.

5. Exceeds our expectations by anticipating and responding   1   2   3   4   5
   to our department's needs before they are verbalized.

6. Briefly describe below what you need from this supplier that you're not receiving.

Supplier number 2...

NEVER   ALWAYS

1. Makes decisions in light of our department's stated needs.   1   2   3   4   5

2. Asks our department what we need or want on a regular basis... 1   2   3   4   5

3. ... and they listen, sincerely, to understand our needs.   1   2   3   4   5

4. Responds to our department's requests and identified needs   1   2   3   4   5
   routinely meeting our predetermined expectations.

5. Exceeds our expectations by anticipating and responding   1   2   3   4   5
   to our department's needs before they are verbalized.

6. Briefly describe below what you need from this supplier that you're not receiving.

Supplier number 3...

NEVER   ALWAYS

1. Makes decisions in light of our department's stated needs.   1   2   3   4   5

2. Asks our department what we need or want on a regular basis... 1   2   3   4   5

3. ... and they listen, sincerely, to understand our needs.   1   2   3   4   5

4. Responds to our department's requests and identified needs   1   2   3   4   5
   routinely meeting our predetermined expectations.

5. Exceeds our expectations by anticipating and responding   1   2   3   4   5
   to our department's needs before they are verbalized.

6. Briefly describe below what you need from this supplier that you're not receiving.

Exhibit 3.10 continued

Feedback for Senior Management

A customer _receives_ and a supplier _provides_ materials, services, or information. Senior and middle managers are both customers and suppliers to each other at different times. For example, a middle manager needing a new piece of equipment for their department will supply their senior manager with the justification of need. The supplied information might be physician requests, patient survey feedback, or an analysis of the potential return on investment. As the senior manager takes the information, analyzes it, defends it, and budgets for it, they transition from a customer to a supplier of (1) a denial or (2) good news and equipment to the middle manager. Unlike some departments, such as human resources (usually a supplier) and patients (almost always customers), managers and their direct reports constantly exchange these roles.

As a customer of senior management, what do you need and want from them? What specific services, actions, or outcomes could they offer you that will help you perform your job successfully? The options below have been left open, intentionally, but some examples might be: communication, clear directions, or input to decisions. Please list the 5 expectations that are most important to you and then determine if your senior manager has met, not met, or exceeded your expectations. _If you mark the "Not Met" box, you must describe a target for improvement, i.e., define the behavior they would have to demonstrate in order to meet your expectations. Please be specific._

The most important services my senior manager can provide which will help me be an effective manager are...

	NOT MET	MET	EXCEEDED
1.	☐	☐	☐
2.	☐	☐	☐
3.	☐	☐	☐
4.	☐	☐	☐
5.	☐	☐	☐

Exhibit 3.11 Feedback for Senior Management

Tally of Participating Hospitals: Feedback for Senior Management

The most important services my senior manager can provide which will help me be an effective manager are...	Not Met	Met	Exceed	Total	
1. Communication (clear/assertive) • Listening	36	58	26	120	94%
2. Leadership • Clear direction • Goals • Vision • Priorities	28	37	24	89	70%
3. Empowers • Backs up decisions • Input to decisions	16	40	14	70	55%
4. Supportive • Understands my department • Respect	19	28	14	61	48%
5. Feedback • Evaluation • Reward • Recognition	27	13	11	51	40%
6. Accessibility • Availability • Involvement	16	18	10	44	
7. Additional resources • Benefits • Budget	11	9	10	30	
8. Development • Training • Professional growth/advancement	9	12	5	26	
9. Honest • Fair • Consistent • Equal treatment	7	4	6	17	
10. Positive work environment	-	2	2	4	
11. Innovative • Creative • Encourages new ideas • Positive	1	1	2	4	
12. Positive role model • Open mind • Coach • Mentor	-	3	1	4	
13. Evaluates programs/procedures • Eliminates or improves	1	1	1	3	
14. Knowledgeable • Conscientious • Competent • Dependable	1	1	1	3	
15. Feeling pride and respect for administration	-	2	-	2	
16. Confidentiality • Trust	1	1	-	2	
17. Proactive • Act rather than react	2	-	-	2	
18. People skills	-	-	1	1	
19. Visibility on other shifts	1	-	-	1	
128 surveys returned TOTALS	176	230	128	534	

Exhibit 3.12 Feedback for Senior Management Results

Observation. It's so simple, it's easy to forget, but a lot of good information can be gained from just watching. Observation, as a data collection technique, can save teams a lot of time by reducing and concentrating the data collection workload. An experience gained by a performance improvement team illustrates the point. The team was brought together to study the problem of the delays in the cafeteria. The line was so long that it took 30 minutes just to get and pay for food. Half-hour meal periods were extended as long as 1 hour and it was affecting patient care, employee satisfaction, and budget performance. A cost-benefit analysis was conducted, and the team was assigned to the task.

Of course, everyone knew what the root cause of the problem was—that everyone went to lunch at the same time, and a bottleneck was created. Wrong! Everyone assumed that was the root cause, and some even applied a solution, sending people to lunch as early as 10:45 AM and as late as 2:30 PM. But the line persisted. On the very first meeting, the team decided, after their attempts at flowcharting failed, to send a team representative to the cafeteria during peak hours to observe. This person was there to watch and experience, and did he ever.

The first thing he observed was that the cups were stored on the far side of the soda dispenser. This meant people had to step out of line to get a cup and then butt back into (a hostile) line to get their sodas. He asked the team leader if a fix could be made this early in the problem-solving process. Warning the team member not to rush to solution, the leader said, "Sure, it's probably not the root cause of the problem, but go ahead and fix it," thinking it would be helpful in clarifying what data should be collected. Well, to everyone's surprise, the cups were moved and the line disappeared. Poof. And while the team member was sitting and observing, he noticed that everyone was throwing away their pickle relish garnish. When he suggested to the cafeteria manager that they have a bowl of garnish available rather than putting one on every sandwich and entree, the manager was only too happy to comply since one full-time person was devoted to this task. An average of 2.2 people per day reached for the pickle relish garnish, and the garnish guru was reassigned.

It's a simple case study but also a compelling example of how simple observation can clear away a lot of junk and clarify what is really important. Sometimes, it is the data collection, and, other times, it clarifies additional data to be collected.

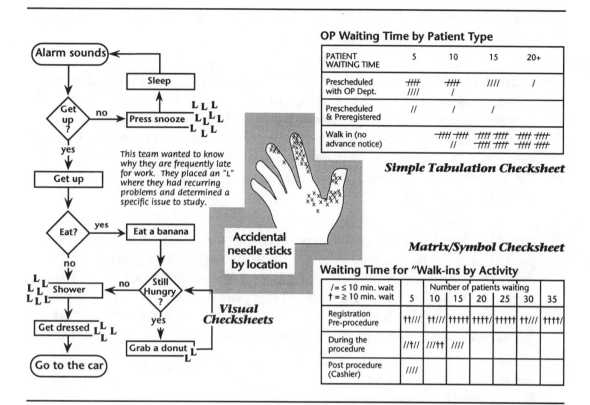

Figure 3.4 Checksheet Examples

Checksheets. The last method of data collection we'll discuss is checksheets. A tool with a dual agenda, checksheets can be used to collect data and display data in a meaningful and easy-to-understand format. They can be used any time a perception needs to be backed up with hard data. Because the end result is always an illustration of some sort, they are particularly helpful when selling an idea or a solution to an audience who is unfamiliar with the issues and data (e.g., physicians, MCOs, senior management). From a team—natural work team or cross-functional team—point of view, the greatest advantage of a checksheet is that several people can collect data simultaneously using a standardized form and then combine their feedback on a single form for presentation and analysis. Since few of us want to give up our day job for data collection, it's a way of sharing the work.

There are several different kinds of checksheets and they are all demonstrated in the examples in Figure 3.4.

- **Simple tabulation checksheets** - This is the checksheet most of us have used. Many of us, sitting in school lecture halls, have made a hatch mark or two (*####*) keeping track of how many times the professor said the nonword "UH." It's also been used by outpatient departments to keep track of patients who come in without appointments. The technique is simple but effective.

- **Visual checksheets** - Visual checksheets inspire creativity and the more creative, the better. As you can see in Figure 3.4, a flowchart can be turned into a checksheet by applying the multivoting technique, and a picture of a hand can become a teaching tool for infection control simply by highlighting where people most often stick themselves. Virtually anything can be turned into a checksheet to depict a situation visually.

- **Matrix checksheets** - While these checksheets are a little more complex, they can provide a lot of useful information in a glance. In the example, the matrix collects data from two vantage points: (1) the number of patients waiting and (2) the part of the process for which they are waiting. At a glance, it's easy to see that the majority of walk-in patients are waiting during the registration/pre-procedure period.

- **Symbol checksheets** - On symbol checksheets, symbols are added to give additional information. In the example, the symbol (/) indicates that the patient waited less than 10 minutes. The symbol (†) indicates a wait of 10 minutes or longer. Looking at the checksheet, it's easy to see that not only are more of the walk-in patients waiting at the registration point, but they are waiting longer periods of time as well. It's a lot of information that can be easily presented and easily understood by any audience.

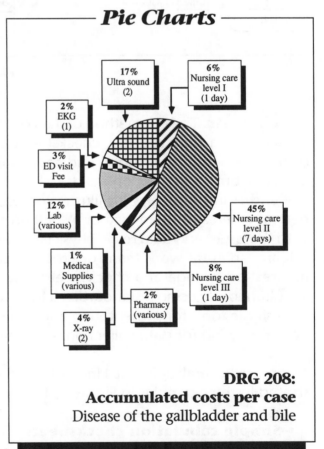

Pie Charts

DRG 208:
Accumulated costs per case
Disease of the gallbladder and bile

Displaying Data for Presentation

A discussion about data collection would be incomplete without a section on presentation. All of us, at some point in our careers, have been presented

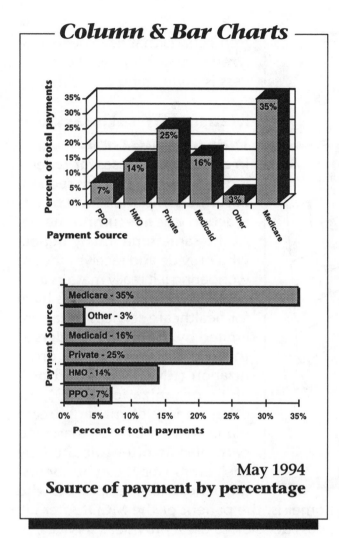

Column & Bar Charts

Payment Source

May 1994
Source of payment by percentage

with a page of data—numbers. And most of us are uncomfortable in this situation. Think about why we collect data. We want to convince someone or some group that something significant is occurring. We want to sell them on an idea. Therefore, it has to be easy. It has to be clear, concise, brief, and succinct. The old adage, "A picture is worth a thousand words," applies here perfectly because people are more likely to accept theories and ideas that they understand. And they are more likely to understand a concept they have visualized. If a checksheet isn't appropriate, here are three other ways to display data for presentation. As you look at the displays, think about what it would be like if you had to describe what you see, in words, instead of pictures.

Pie Charts. Pie charts provide a way to display 100% of the data as well as individual percentages and their relationship to the total. Pie charts are great standalone charts because they require little or no explanation. There's also a lot you can do artistically with a pie chart to jazz up a presentation with colors, labels, and detached slices of the pie.

Column and Bar Charts. These types of charts allow comparisons among data and sometimes show a pattern. Pareto diagrams and histograms are examples of column charts. In both cases, the goal is to find a significant pattern or trend that will enable a prediction or confidence, that if "x" process continues, "y" outcome will occur. They are excellent for assessment and analysis, which will be discussed in more depth in the next chapter.

Run or Trend Charts. These well-known monitoring displays illustrate performance results over time. They are extremely useful for studying processes and the performance of the process over time. Control charts are

Run/Trend Charts

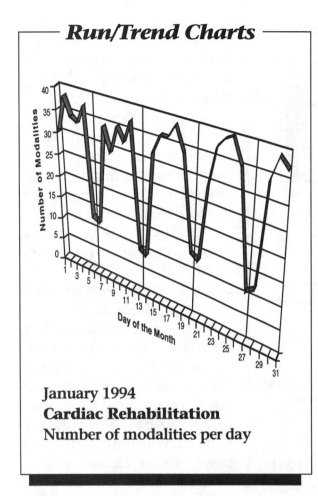

January 1994
Cardiac Rehabilitation
Number of modalities per day

trend charts that have been analyzed to assess how well the process is performing over time.

Measuring satisfaction: Will anyone care?

In all of the processes for collecting data reviewed in this section, customers and their level of satisfaction was a recurring theme. At the same time, many people who provide and receive care are wondering if it really matters anymore. The choices patients have for healthcare services today are limited by the list of providers in their health maintenance organization (HMO), preferred provider organization (PPO), or other variety of managed care plan. Their choice of managed care plan is often dictated by their employer. It can be confusing to healthcare employees who may wonder who their real customer is, the patient or the MCO. After all, it's the MCO that makes the business decision to use a provider's services, or not, to pay for the service, or not.

Despite this reality, the answer to the question is a firm "yes." Clearly, in immature managed care markets, there is a heavy lean toward money being the primary factor considered by managed care providers and by businesses purchasing healthcare coverage for their employees. However, in the more mature markets of California and Minnesota, there is a lot more discussion and attention being paid to patient satisfaction (is the system user-friendly and efficient), clinical outcomes (are patients receiving quality care), and their MCOs' overall ability to contain costs.

As more data become available to the American public, MCOs will be able to make more informed decisions regarding which facility actually delivers the highest quality care and which organization can do so at the most reasonable cost, and purchasers of healthcare—businesses and individuals—will be able to use outcome data to influence the purchase of the healthcare insurance of their choice.

Notes

1. Joint Commission on Accreditation of Healthcare Organizations, *Accreditation Manual for Hospitals: Volume II* (Oakbrook Terrace, IL: Joint Commission, 1994), 18.

2. J. Lawthers and P. Wood, In Search of Psychiatric Performance Measures, *Clinical Performance and Quality Health Care* 4, no. 1 (1996), 38–40.

3. Joint Commission, *News Release* (January 23, 1996), 1–3.

4. Joint Commission, *News Release* (March 5, 1996), 1.

5. Joint Commission, *Accreditation Manual for Hospitals* (1996), 190.

6. Joint Commission, *Accreditation Manual for Hospitals* (1994), 18.

Recommended Reading

Brazzoli, F. 1995. Repositories promise to quench growing thirst for health data. *Health Data Management.* October: 50–56.

Deming, W.E. 1986. *Out of Crisis.* Cambridge, MA: MIT Press.

Joint Commission IMS and Maryland QIP: A tale of two indicator systems. 1996. *Quality Management Update.* January 10: 5–8.

Kennedy, M. 1995–6. Strategic performance measurement systems: Next step after dashboards. *The Quality Letter for Healthcare Leaders.* December 95–January 96: 2–21.

Lau, L. et al. 1996. Quality assessment and patient participation in care by means of a touch-screen computer. *Clinical Performance and Quality Health Care.* January–February–March: 10–13.

Montague, J. 1994. Do-it-yourself outcomes. *Hospitals & Health Networks.* July 5: 42–44.

Palmer, R. 1996. Measuring clinical performance to provide information for quality improvement. *Quality Management in Health Care.* Winter: 1–6.

Pehrson, G. 1994. Using care process models to improve quality while controlling cost. *The Quality Letter for Healthcare Leaders.* April: 24–27.

Smith, M. 1994. Emerging trends and issues for healthcare information management. In *Guide to Effective Health Care Information and Management Systems.* Chicago: Healthcare Information and Management Systems Society, 11–16.

Spath, P. 1995. To sample or not to sample? *Hospital Case Management.* August: 128–130.

Using patient input in a cycle for performance improvement. 1995. *The Joint Commission Journal on Quality Improvement.* February: 87–96.

Zablocki, E. 1996. Health systems go beyond satisfaction to win customer loyalty. *The Quality Letter for Healthcare Leaders.* April: 2–8.

TORTURE
THE DATA LONG
ENOUGH AND THEY
WILL CONFESS TO
ANYTHING

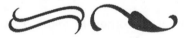

- ANONYMOUS

4. ASSESSMENT

Integrated Quality Management

Analyze and Assess

Before delving into this subject, some definitions might be helpful:

- *Assess* to judge or evaluate
- *Analyze* to resolve into its important parts; study critically

Why is a distinction useful? Because if time is taken to study and analyze an outcome, process, or cost carefully and properly, assessment of how well things are going will be a lot easier.

A dear friend and colleague, George Labovitz, spoke once of performance management in terms of bowling. He said, in his own inimitable way, that some performance management systems were like bowling with a curtain in front of the pins. You roll the ball, hear pins falling, but can see nothing. The bowler yells to the pinsetter, "How am I doing," and a voice comes back, "I'll tell you at your annual merit evaluation."

There are countless performance management systems available today. Some are subjective and can be swayed easily by the personalities of the evaluators. Most of us do not want to be evaluated by that type of system, and in fact, it's a lot harder for the evaluator as well. The easiest, and best, assessment systems are the ones that set an expected, measurable outcome that is desired. Actual performance is then measured against that outcome and compared. It is either met, not met, or exceeded. No subjectivity; no ambiguous language (what does *good* mean anyway?); and, very important, if the individual wants to know what to do to improve, he or she can just read the performance outcomes, process, and productivity standards. There are no surprises, no "I gotcha." And individuals can self-assess at any point in time to know how well they are doing.

Several examples of this type of performance assessment system are shown on the following pages, and, by now, they should be looking familiar to readers. One of the primary benefits of the **Indicator Development Worksheet** is that as standards and indicators are being designed, the as-

111

sessment system is simultaneously being created. An example of this is shown in Exhibit 4.1, **Indicator Assessment Plan for Laparoscopy**. For each outcome, process, and cost related to labor time, there is an opportunity to rate performance: not met, met, or exceeded. The very same standards that were designed to facilitate customer expectations can now be used to evaluate and assess performance results. Briefly, when the assessment is completed, it will reveal the following:

- Were the **outcomes** achieved? The big question and the one that has always been asked, and always will be asked, because it is the bottom line. Were clinical goals met? Were customers satisfied? How do we compare to others? How do we compare to our own past performance?

- Did the **process** work and was it followed? An unmet outcome usually means that (1) the process is broken, inefficient, or ineffective, or (2) the process is terrific, but it's not being followed. Note that this part of the assessment tool can be used for a criteria-based performance evaluation of staff members. In Exhibit 4.6, part of a case study later in the chapter, the detailed approach to the Indicator Assessment Plan creates a clinical path for diabetic ketoacidosis (DKA). It's easy to see in this example how *process indicators* serve a second purpose as performance appraisal standards for caregivers. Once again, that person's clinical performance can be assessed by comparing actual performance to the standard, which is then met, not met, or exceeded.

- Was the process completed within the **cost** constraints of managed care? Is it an affordable process? Is it efficient? In the years to come some organizations will fail to thrive despite great outcomes and effective processes because they are simply not affordable.

Several examples follow in Exhibits 4.2 through 4.6. As results are assessed and analyzed throughout this chapter, keep in mind that the results are not just about clinical and service outcomes, but process and cost as well.

Baseline Information

When assessing any kind of data, baseline information is required for several reasons. One, it can identify and document where you were at the beginning of the process or project. Two, sometimes a problem seems enormous because we are still in the middle of it, flinching in pain. Data are a lot less emotional than human beings and a lot better at describing the enormity of an issue. Three, assumptions can lead us off in the wrong direction, and data can verify if, in fact, our assumptions are valid.

Care or Service Outcome Indicators	Performance or Process Indicators	Financial Indicators
Care (clinical and satisfaction) or service results	Recommended process and employee responsibilities	Necessary or avoidable cost

Laparoscopy

Strategic Priority: *Become the ambulatory surgery provider of choice in the community.*
Performance Improvement Priority: *Increase volume of ambulatory surgical procedures while maintaining costs.*

ASSESSMENT
- **Baseline physiologic parameters established**
  Not Met ☐ Met ☐ Exceeded ☐
- **Ongoing monitoring of changes in parameters**
  Not Met ☐ Met ☐ Exceeded ☐

IVs
- **Proper healing without developing an infection from the IV system**
  Not Met ☐ Met ☐ Exceeded ☐
- **Administration of fluids**
  Not Met ☐ Met ☐ Exceeded ☐

DRESSINGS
- **Prevention of infection**
  Not Met ☐ Met ☐ Exceeded ☐
- **Aid wound healings**
  Not Met ☐ Met ☐ Exceeded ☐

TEACHING
- **Patient and/or family are able to verbalize knowledge of patient's care plan**
  Not Met ☐ Met ☐ Exceeded ☐
- **Written discharge plan complete**
  Not Met ☐ Met ☐ Exceeded ☐

Preoperative visit (2–5 days prior to surgery):
- Neuro checks (305.3)
- Breath/bowel sounds (305.4)
- Preop teaching (301.4)
- TPR and B/P (305.2)
- History & Physical
- Blood tests

Not Met ☐ Met ☐ Exceeded ☐ — **30 minutes**
Not Met ☐ Met ☐ Exceeded ☐

Admission, preoperative monitoring:
- Preop teaching (301.4)
- With piggyback (444.13)
- IV start (444.14)
- With meds (444.11)

Not Met ☐ Met ☐ Exceeded ☐ — **20 minutes**
Not Met ☐ Met ☐ Exceeded ☐

Intraoperative phase 1 hour (1 nurse:1 patient):
Not Met ☐ Met ☐ Exceeded ☐ — **60 minutes**
Not Met ☐ Met ☐ Exceeded ☐

1st stage recovery 1 hour (1 nurse:1 patient):
Not Met ☐ Met ☐ Exceeded ☐ — **60 minutes**
Not Met ☐ Met ☐ Exceeded ☐

2nd stage recovery 1 hour (1 nurse:4 patients):
Not Met ☐ Met ☐ Exceeded ☐ — **15 minutes**
Not Met ☐ Met ☐ Exceeded ☐

3rd stage recovery/Discharge instructions and postop teaching 1 hour (1 nurse:4 patients):
- Activity goals and limitations (Procedure 444.10)
- Dressing change (Procedure 331.1)
- Medication instructions (Procedure 432.5)
- Nutrition plan (Procedure 421.3)

Not Met ☐ Met ☐ Exceeded ☐ — **15 minutes**
Not Met ☐ Met ☐ Exceeded ☐

Average total procedure time: 3.3 hours
Not Met ☐ Met ☐ Exceeded ☐

Indicator Assessment Plan

Exhibit 4.1 Indicator Assessment Plan for Laparoscopy

Contributed by: Daniel Gilbert, Assistant Administrator for Human Resources • Bradley Memorial Hospital, Cleveland, Tennessee.

Indicator Assessment Plan

Strategic Priority: To be competitive in a managed care market while maintaining both internal and external customer focus.

Performance Improvement Priority: Managers will manage their respective areas appropriately and effectively.

Care or Service Outcome Indicators Care (clinical and satisfaction) or service results	Performance or Process Indicators Recommended process and employee responsibilities	Financial Indicators Necessary or avoidable cost
Standard: All managers will complete the entire curriculum of Bradley University. *Indicators:* 1. All current managers will complete the entire curriculum within one year. Not Met □ Met □ Exceeded □ 2. All new managers must complete the core courses within six months of hire or promotion and the management courses within one year of hire or promotion. Not Met □ Met □ Exceeded □ 3. Upon completion of the program, each participant will demonstrate knowledge of course content and subject matter for each class offering. Not Met □ Met □ Exceeded □	*Standard:* Participants will meet the learning objectives of each of the 18 individual Bradley U. courses. *Indicators:* Participants will: (examples from three of the courses) 1. Identify and use various CQI tools and appropriate indicators for use (CQI course). Not Met □ Met □ Exceeded □ 2. Recognize common budgeting strategies (Financial Management course). Not Met □ Met □ Exceeded □ 3. Demonstrate proficiency in conducting an interview and job offer (Interview and Selection Techniques course). Not Met □ Met □ Exceeded □	*Standard: Participants will use skills obtained to manage their respective areas appropriately and effectively.* *Indicators:* 1. Improve processes to increase user/customer satisfaction by 10 points. Not Met □ Met □ Exceeded □ 2. Department expense budget standards will be met within 5% of target. Not Met □ Met □ Exceeded □ 3. Decrease the turnover rate for employees in their 90-day introductory period from 5% to 4%. Not Met □ Met □ Exceeded □

Exhibit 4.2 Assessment Plan: Management Development

Contributed by: Rebecca Marinos, RN, MSN, CCRN • Columbia Medical Center, Brazos Valley, College Station, Texas.

Care or Service Outcome Indicators Care (clinical and satisfaction) or service results	**Performance or Process Indicators** Recommended process and employee responsibilities	**Financial Indicators** Necessary or avoidable cost
Strategic Priority: Critical Care **Performance Improvement Priority:** *Family Support*		
Standard: Family of critically ill patient will receive emotional support. Indicator: Family will be able to verbalize emotional needs. Not Met ☐ Met ☐ Exceeded ☐	Standard: Each nurse will evaluate the family's response to crisis situation. Indicator: Each nurse will document family's response in the patient's record. Not Met ☐ Met ☐ Exceeded ☐	Standard: Resources will be available and utilized appropriately. Indicator: Ongoing Not Met ☐ Met ☐ Exceeded ☐
IA: Head injury patient/family teaching Standard: Each patient/family will receive information related to his/her condition and care of that condition. Indicator: Each patient/family will be able to verbalize knowledge of head trauma, medications, and rehabilitation plans. Not Met ☐ Met ☐ Exceeded ☐	Standard: Each nurse will evaluate the patient's and family's response and outcomes. Indicator: Each nurse will document knowledge status in the patient's record. Not Met ☐ Met ☐ Exceeded ☐	Standard: Resources will be available and utilized appropriately. Indicator: 1 hour (average) Not Met ☐ Met ☐ Exceeded ☐
IA: Wound care Standard: Each patient will receive appropriate wound care. Indicator: Wound will heal without evidence of complication. Not Met ☐ Met ☐ Exceeded ☐	• Initial assessment of wound: Size in cm, color, shape, drainage, depth, cause if known • Consultation with MD re frequency and type of wound care • Patient Instruction • Premedicate with analgesics • Perform wound care • Document care/condition of wound Not Met ☐ Met ☐ Exceeded ☐	Indicator: 1 hour, 55 min. Not Met ☐ Met ☐ Exceeded ☐
IA: Early postoperative ambulation for abdominal surgery Standard: Each patient will begin ambulation first postoperative day. Indicator: Patient is able to ambulate one day after abdominal surgery. Not Met ☐ Met ☐ Exceeded ☐	• Obtain MD order for ambulation one day post procedure • Patient instruction • Secure invasive lines • Sit patient on side of bed • Ambulate to chair Not Met ☐ Met ☐ Exceeded ☐	Indicator: 45 minutes total Not Met ☐ Met ☐ Exceeded ☐

Indicator Assessment Plan

Exhibit 4.3 Assessment Plan for Critical Care

Contributed by: Lori Brown, Data Processing Manager • St. Francis Medical Center, Grand Island, Nebraska.

Care or Service **Outcome** Indicators	Performance or **Process** Indicators	**Financial Indicators**
Care (clinical and satisfaction) or service results	Recommended process and employee responsibilities	Necessary or avoidable cost

Strategic Priority: *Information Systems*
Performance Improvement Priority: *Operations*

Standard:
Computer system access is available.

Indicator:
The computer will be available for all users 95% of the time.

Completion date: 12/1

Not Met ☐   Met ☐   Exceeded ☐

Data Processing Manager Responsibilities:

1. *Make sure all device problems and software problems are addressed within 1/2 hour.*   30 minutes, plus actual problem time

2. *Make sure all updates are loaded in a timely fashion and users notified immediately when completed.*   Variable

3. *Complete daily backups to ensure security.*   3 hours

4. *Keep a downtime log of detailed causes of downtime.*   15 minutes

5. *Monitor downtime log to prevent problems occurring again.*   30 minutes

6. *Provide trouble shooting maintenance procedures for users on a rotating basis.*   30 minutes

7. *Schedule updates and preventive maintenance to Avions in the same time frame when possible.*   As requested

Not Met ☐   Met ☐   Exceeded ☐   Not Met ☐   Met ☐   Exceeded ☐

Indicator Assessment Plan

Exhibit 4.4 Assessment Plan: Information Systems

Contributed by: Vaughn Minton, Information Systems Director • St. Francis Medical Center, Grand Island, Nebraska.

Care or Service Outcome Indicators Care (clinical and satisfaction) or service results	**Performance or Process Indicators** Recommended process and employee responsibilities	**Financial Indicators** Necessary or avoidable cost

Strategic Priority: *Information Systems*
Performance Improvement Priority: *Analyst support*

Data Processing Manager Responsibilities:

<u>Standard:</u>
Develop ongoing "refresher" training courses for all supported applications.

<u>Indicator:</u>
100% of users interviewed by department director will have satisfactory or better results.

<u>Completion date:</u> *6/30*

Not Met ❑   Met ❑   Exceeded ❑

1. *Survey users to identify key areas for training (no later than 12/1).*
   Not Met ❑   Met ❑   Exceeded ❑

2. *Create at least one IADAT training tape for each application in "Live status" as of Oct. 1.*
   Not Met ❑   Met ❑   Exceeded ❑

3. *Create supporting documentation of the IADAT training tapes (see step #2).*
   Not Met ❑   Met ❑   Exceeded ❑

4. *Develop and maintain catalog of training tapes.*
   Not Met ❑   Met ❑   Exceeded ❑

5. *Notify users via e-mail (Meditech) that training tapes are available.*
   Not Met ❑   Met ❑   Exceeded ❑

- *4 hours per analyst (20 hours total)*
  Not Met ❑ Met ❑ Exceeded ❑

- *10 hours per IADAT tape (25 tapes @ 10 hours/tape = 250 hrs)*
  Not Met ❑ Met ❑ Exceeded ❑

- *8 hrs per IADAT tape (25 tapes @ 8 hours/ tape = 200 hrs)*
  Not Met ❑ Met ❑ Exceeded ❑

- *15 minutes per tape (25 tapes @ 15 min/ tape = 3 hours)*
  Not Met ❑ Met ❑ Exceeded ❑

Indicator Assessment Plan

Exhibit 4.5 Assessment Plan: Information Analyst Support

Contributed by: Pamela Hall, RN, MBA, Quality Improvement Director • Stephens County Hospital, Toccoa, Georgia.

Care or Service Outcome Indicators Care (clinical and satisfaction) or service results	Performance or Process Indicators Recommended process and employee responsibilities	Financial Indicators Necessary or avoidable cost
Strategic Priority: Improve and expand diabetic treatment program. **Performance Improvement Priority: Improve clinical outcomes while maintaining or reducing costs.**		*Costs*
Diabetic Ketoacidosis (DKA): Day 1	*Diagnostics*	
The patient's electrolyte, acid-base balance and dehydration will be corrected.	If glucose > 250 in presence of mental status changes, the following will be done: ABGs, EKG, SMA 22, urine or serum ketones.	Cost of test
	Repeat SMA 6 in 4 hours.	Cost of test
	Repeat ABGs in 1 hour if pH < 7.2.	Cost of test
	Physician to rule/out underlying diagnoses which may have contributed to development of DKA.	1 hr. physician time, cost of tests
	Medications	
	Regular insulin 10 units IV push	Medication cost
	Begin insulin drip of regular insulin 20 units in 100cc D_5 administered at ___ cc/hr (to achieve administration of insulin 5-7 units/hr with 20-30 cc/hr recommended).	Medication cost plus .25 hours staff time
	Nursing to notify physician 2 hours post insulin drip initiation, if Accuchek levels have not fallen 50-100 mg/hr	.25 hours
	Decrease insulin rate by 1/2 when the Accuchek reaches 250.	.25 hours
	Continue insulin drip until ketones are negative and patient is on sliding scale insulin.	Medication cost plus .5 hours staff time
	If patient is producing urine and there are no signs of severe hyperkalemia, add KCL 20 meq to second liter of IV fluids.	Medication cost plus .25 hours
	Continue KCL infusion thereafter, if serum K not elevated.	Medication cost plus .25 hours
	Physician to consider $NaHCO_3$ based on pH	No cost
	Begin sliding scale insulin before stopping IV insulin drip.	Medication cost plus .25 hours
	Treatments	
	Fingerstick glucose every 1 hour for 6 hours, then every 2 hours	Accuchek cost plus 1.5 hours
	Foley for no urine output	Foley tray cost plus .5 hours
	Intake and output	1.0 hours of staff time
	Vital signs every 1 hour for two times, then every 2 hours	.75 hours of staff time
	Weight (ask if unable to obtain)	.1 hours of staff time
	Nasogastric tube if in a coma or severe vomiting	NG supplies, 24-hr suction, .5 hrs
	Assess mental status every 2 hours.	.5 hours of staff time
	Urine ketones with every voiding or every 4 hrs with Foley catheter	Supply cost plus .5 hours

(Continues)

Indicator Assessment Plan

Exhibit 4.6 Assessment Plan: Diabetic Ketoacidosis

Care or Service Outcome Indicators Care (clinical and satisfaction) or service results	Performance or Process Indicators Recommended process and employee responsibilities	Financial Indicators Necessary or avoidable cost
DKA: Day 1 (continued)		
	Nutrition Patient should be NPO.	No cost
Education and discharge planning will begin.	*Education/Discharge Planning* Assess for cause of DKA. Assess knowledge of diabetic diet. Assess financial resources for purchase of diabetic supplies post-discharge. Assess family support postdischarge. Document assessment and make appropriate referrals to Diabetic Educator, Social Services, or Dietitian.	.25 hours .25 hours .25 hours .25 hours .25 hours
DKA: Day 2 The patient will be able to tolerate intake of regular diabetic diet.	*Nutrition* Discontinue NG tube when nausea subsides. The appropriate calorie ADA diet will be initiated.	.25 hours .1 hr (no cost for meal)
	Diagnostics SMA 6 on AM of Day 2 Repeat any abnormal labs from Day 1.	Cost of test Cost of tests
	Treatments Daily weight Vital signs 4 times a day Fingerstick glucose before meals and at bedtime Prevention methods will be taught relative to the cause of DKA. Health activities will be reviewed to prevent DKA. Begin instruction for self-administration of insulin. If previously instructed, review patient administration procedures.	.25 hours staff time .75 hours .75 hours .5 hours .5 hours 1–2 hours
DKA: Day 3 The patient's insulin needs will stabilize. The patient will be knowledgeable of diabetic diet.	*Treatments* Physician will adjust insulin dose to achieve desired blood sugar levels. Assess/review for diet teaching. Followup with additional diabetic-related teaching needs on an out-patient basis or refer to Outpatient Diabetic monthly classes.	Tests, meds, .5 hrs. physician time .5 hours .25 hours for referral, 1–4 hrs for additional teaching

Indicator Assessment Plan

Exhibit 4.6 continued

Baseline data are easy to find. In fact, they are probably sitting on someone's desk at this very minute. Any data that are collected, for any reason, may become baseline information for your next project, as long as they can verify current performance levels. It's important to know where you're coming from as it relates to where you're going.

A case study. The Stephens County Hospital example in Exhibit 4.6 demonstrates the value of both baseline and ongoing data assessment. Developed as a clinical path for diabetic ketoacidosis (DKA), the initial goals were aimed at improving clinical quality and reducing costs, and the team members were quite successful at both. In the beginning, they looked at solving individual problems but subsequently developed this critical pathway with the help of several physicians. Duplications were eliminated; functions were standardized; length of stay shortened almost immediately; and costs, with two exceptions, fell within a normal range of variation (Figure 4.1). Most notable, daily outcomes were being met consistently (88% of the time). Two significant factors were (1) the correction of dehydration and electrolyte acid base balance on the first day, resulting in improved quality and lower costs, and (2) increased physician compliance, which grew from 67% in January 1995 to 75% in March, to 88% in September.

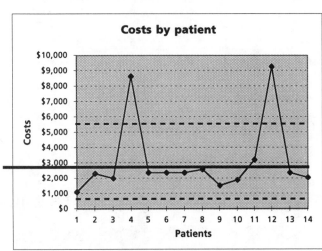

Figure 4.1 Tracking Costs by Patient

Next, in Figure 4.2, comorbidities were studied as a possible cost factor and found that more comorbidities did not necessarily affect the length of stay or the costs. When the two cases were studied as individual cases, the team learned that one patient went to the intensive care unit (ICU) and the other did not follow the recommended critical path. Looking at the cost performance of the remaining patients, it's satisfying to see that their costs are right at, or below, the target goal of $2,800. The fact that these costs were below target means that reimbursement from third-party payers com-

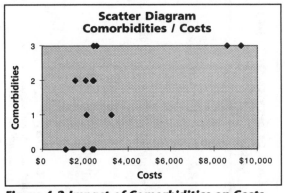

Figure 4.2 Impact of Comorbidities on Costs

ing in would more than cover their costs and leave them in a profitable position for this particular critical pathway. In terms of both outcome and cost performance, it's a great example of what a group of subject matter experts can accomplish by redesigning a process.

It also reinforces the reality that consensus must mean more than a nod of the head. It's an agreement to change behavior in order to attain better results. Measures hold people accountable to the new behavior and indicate whether or not the new process is working as expected.

Common Causes and Special Causes

If it normally takes 15 minutes to drive to work, but one day it takes an hour, would you change the process you use to go to work? Probably not. If it happens over and over again (a recurring problem or *common cause*), however, you might begin to think, "Hey, this is not an accident or a rare occurrence, this is how it's going to be, and it's time to find another route." The same premise holds for any process. If there is a one-time blip (sometimes called a *special cause*), you would want to be able to predict, avoid, prevent, even fix. But you wouldn't want to change the system or process on the basis of so little information. The exception would be if it was a *sentinel event*, one with consequences so severe that intensive assessment is required, and not just at the site of the incident. You can be sure that after the wrong foot was amputated from a man at a Florida hospital, every hospital in the nation wondered, "Do we have a plan in place to prevent this from happening in our hospital?" On the other hand, if it's a good special cause—showing a performance level far better than the norm—you would definitely want to study what's going on, reward those involved, and see if that special cause success could be replicated.

Case study. The example in Figure 4.3 is from an emergency department (ED) team. Their original charge was to reduce the waiting time in the ED; however, when the team convened and flowcharted their process, they decided that the delays were caused by the lack of an ICU bed, not ED processes. The team brought on ICU representatives and discovered that it wasn't an ICU problem, it was a patient-flow problem. They would happily receive ED patients sooner if only they could find a bed on the floor. After detailed interviewing and discussion with supervisors regarding why beds on the floor were never available, team members discovered a recurring problem. Patients were being discharged at 9:00 AM, and at 7:00 PM, they were still there! The newly narrowed and focused problem was late discharges, and the team began to collect data.

The ICU nurse manager was nervous. First, she had lived through a horrendous May that required daily bed patrol duties to move patients in and out of ICU. Second, in July, she had had to cover the house for the regular supervisor who was recuperating from surgery. Frustrated by the bed availability problem, she had been sending patients home in taxi cabs (with permission from family, physician, and patient) at the hospital's expense. She rationalized (correctly) that every time the ED was backed up and an ambulance had to bypass the hospital to go to another ED, revenue was going along with it. Nonetheless, she feared that she would be caught. Just as she feared, she was caught. Then, surprisingly, she was rewarded for her contribution to solving the problem. Her decisions in July produced that big dip in late discharges and provided a new process that was adopted as a standard operating procedure and offered to every patient in need. Ultimately, as the statistical process control chart shows, the late discharges were reduced, patients flowed out of ICU, and the ED had more options for assigning their patients.

The statistical process control chart shows that because of a change in the system (a group of processes) for discharging patients, team members were able to achieve a *sustained* improvement in their performance results. This achievement reinforced a well-known theory of W. Edwards Deming that reducing variation in and, thus, improving processes is the most reliable way to achieve and sustain improvements.[1] (The late Dr. Deming was an internationally renowned American consultant who was sent to Japan to teach the Japanese management and who revolutionized worldwide management of quality and productivity.) Given the substantial *avoidable* cost of quality—lost business from patients who bypassed the overflowing ED, lost revenue from beds that were occupied by nonpaying discharged patients, wasted staff time, etc.—whatever time was spent on teamwork and data analysis more than paid for itself.

Trends and Patterns

Two other important indicators that are helpful in assessing and analyzing data are *trends* and *patterns*. In the statistical process control chart (Figure 4.3), there were trends (within the control limits), but not repeating patterns. Why are trends and patterns important? For one, trends indicate recurring problems. Recurring problems eat up time and money but *can be fixed by changing the process or system*. For another, trends and patterns visually display what is occurring with data. When numberphobics are given a page full of statistics, their eyes tend to glaze over. The same data placed in a graph or pie chart becomes a lot easier to analyze. In the process of analyzing data for evaluation purposes, trends and patterns play an important role in both providing clues and confirming or disproving assumptions.

In addition to the control chart, the Pareto diagram is a reliable visual display of the 80-20 Rule (a.k.a. the Pareto Principle). Named after Vilfredo

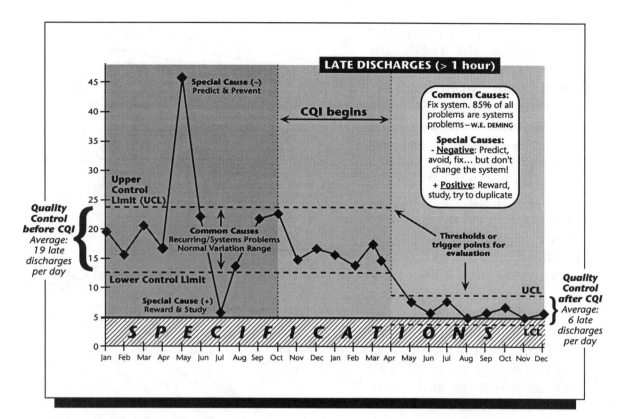

Specifications
(a.k.a: Standards, indicators, goals, targets, wishes)

- Indicates the level of **performance you need** and **want**.

- Based on what is required by **employees**, the **customer**, and the **process** itself.

- Data collection and analysis should indicate if the process is **performing as it should**.

- **Example**: Zero incidents of lost dentures. Zero dollars paid.

Control Limits
(a.k.a: Norms, thresholds, normal range of variation)

- Indicates how the process **usually performs.**

- **Calculated** using historical data of the process and a mathematical formula (consult an expert).

- Data collection and analysis should indicate if **process** is doing **something unusual** (out of control?).

- **Example**: Decrease incidents of lost dentures and dollars paid by a minimum of 2% by date.

Figure 4.3 Statistical Process Control Chart Showing Common Causes, Special Causes, and Normal Variation

Pareto, an Italian economist who lived in the 1800s, the principle "suggests that most effects come from relatively few causes; that is, 80% of the effects come from 20% of the possible causes."[2] For example, 80% of the wealth might be held by 20% of the population, or 80% of our time is spent on only 20% of the duties listed on our job description, or 80% of the beer is drunk by only 20% of the beer drinkers. The more this theory has been tested, the more it has been found to hold true. People refer to and rely heavily on Pareto's 80-20 rule to prioritize and focus their attention and energy.

Continuing with the last case study, the two examples of Pareto diagrams shown in Figure 4.4 are some of the data

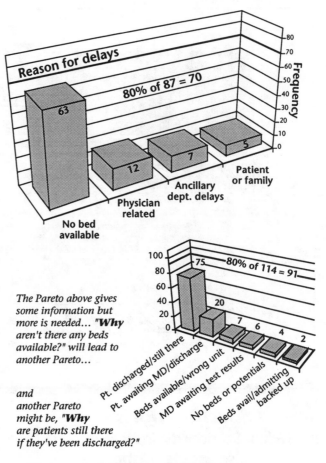

*The Pareto above gives some information but more is needed... "**Why** aren't there any beds available?" will lead to another Pareto...*

*and another Pareto might be, "**Why** are patients still there if they've been discharged?"*

Figure 4.4 Pareto Diagrams

that were analyzed to identify and prioritize a root cause of the "late discharge" problem. Typically, Pareto diagrams respond to who, what, where, when, why, and how questions. Here, the first question is, "What is the reason for the delay?" Even though it's not quite a Pareto (80%), it shows, clearly, that the lack of bed availability is a major cause, which led to another Pareto, "Why aren't there any beds available?" and a third, "Why are patients still there if they have been discharged?" Each time, the Pareto is being used to dig deeper and deeper into the issue to zero in on the root cause of the problem. In some cases, it is reinforcing an assumption, and, in others, it is surprising users by proving the assumption incorrect.

The value of the 80-20 rule cannot be overstated. In general, managed care and other cost constraints are forcing an environment where care providers simply cannot do it all anymore; therefore, prioritizing workload is essential. More specifically to the subject of analysis and assessment, few of us have the time—or the interest—to assess everything, and the 80-20 rule is very helpful in both narrowing down the volume of data to analyze and performing the actual analysis of the data.

Turning Data into Management Information

Most organizations today have data—lots of data. Some are drowning in their data. But that doesn't always mean they have information. It's the analysis, the critical study, and the assessment and evaluation that turn data into information. Today's organizations critically need information for decision making, planning, benchmarking, budgeting, and problem solving. And no one can afford to guess or work from assumptions when the stakes are so high and the constraints so rigid. Thus, as each set of data is analyzed and assessed, it becomes more useful to the manager and more informative.

One last example from the "late discharges" case study will reinforce this point. Team members collected a lot of data, analyzed the data, and discovered that, in fact, the root cause of their problem was the number of patients who were discharged early in the morning but were still there past dinner time. The team prioritized three possible solutions.

1. As patients are discharged, they will be moved to a comfortable and attractive waiting area. Meals will be served and medicines will be given until the patient is picked up by his or her family.

2. Creation of a hospital-owned and operated limousine service. Patients could select as a method of transportation home, or, with physician and family approval, it could be offered to patients as an alternative to being charged for an additional day. Patients in need of assistance upon their arrival at home could utilize the services of the hospital's home health agency to help them get settled.

3. Begin operating the hospital as a hotel. Alert all involved parties that discharge will occur by 11:00 AM. After that time, any patients remaining in their rooms will be charged for an additional day, which would probably not be covered by their insurance.

Solution 3 was ruled out as it was perceived to be too abrasive for the competitive market of the hospital. **Cost-benefit analysis** was applied to the available cost data. (See Exhibit 4.7.) Cost-benefit analysis is a tool used to calculate the return on investment and is invaluable in equalizing solutions for selection. Too many teams pass up excellent solutions because they cost more to implement, without ever looking at the potential return on investment, which may be exponential. In this case, however, the least expensive option also gave a larger ratio of benefits to cost (return on investment). In the limo service option—a derivative of the ICU nurse manager's taxi op-

Option #1 or

Limo Service   **1 year**

PROPOSED SOLUTION OR OPTION   ANALYSIS PERIOD

TANGIBLE COSTS	DOLLAR VALUE	TANGIBLE BENEFITS	DOLLAR VALUE
• Limo/Van lease	$10,000	• Recaptured revenue: 4 rescue squad cases per month @ $25,000 each	$1.2M
• Car expenses and insurance	5,000		
• Driver Salary	20,000		$1,200,000
• Planning	1,500		
• Start-up	3,000		
	$39,500		

INTANGIBLE COSTS	INTANGIBLE BENEFITS
• Patients may go home without enough family support	• Ease bed availability
	• Convenience for staff
• Resistance to the new process by patients, staff, and physicians	• Patients can be home sooner

$$\frac{Benefits}{Costs} = \text{Cost Benefit Ratio}\quad \frac{\$1,200,000}{\$39,500} = 30.4$$

Option #2

Waiting Area   **1 year**

PROPOSED SOLUTION OR OPTION   ANALYSIS PERIOD

TANGIBLE COSTS	DOLLAR VALUE	TANGIBLE BENEFITS	DOLLAR VALUE
• Furniture/TV	$15,000	• Recaptured revenue: 4 rescue squad cases per month @ $25,000 each	$1.2M
• Closing two patient rooms @ 80% occupancy	292,000		
• Staffing	$12,000		$1,200,000
• Desk/Supplies	$3,000		
	$322,000		

INTANGIBLE COSTS	INTANGIBLE BENEFITS
• Patients like being in their own room	• Ease bed availability
• Not private	• Convenience for staff
• Physicians might not support use	• Easy to use and start up

$$\frac{Benefits}{Costs} = \text{Cost Benefit Ratio}\quad \frac{\$1,200,000}{\$322,000} = 3.7$$

Exhibit 4.7 Cost-Benefit Analysis of Possible Solutions

tion—for every dollar spent to run the service, $30.40 would come back in revenue and business. Taking the time to analyze the data and turn it into information made the management decision much easier and even opened up discussion of adding the home health aide, either as a patient charge item or free service.

Financial data are another very important group that can be turned into management information. The **Resource Utilization Report Cards**, Exhibits 4.8 and 4.9, are two examples (one outpatient, one inpatient) of how managers can turn raw data into valuable assessment and evaluation information. In both cases, the reviewer can quickly see volume (activity) levels, acuity-required (classified) hours, and the actual hours of care or service provided. With a few simple calculations—which are shown on the form itself—productivity indexes can be identified, and performance can be evaluated.

Looking closer at Exhibit 4.8, the calculations at the bottom in section "D" show that the rehabilitation department budgeted for 1.0 labor hour of care per modality. The classified, or acuity-required, hours indicated that 1.1 hours, or 10% more time, was needed, given the actual profile of the modalities ordered. Unfortunately, the manager staffed the unit for 1.2 hours per modality (HPM), another 10% more than what was needed and 20% more than what was budgeted. Given the goal of 100% productivity with a

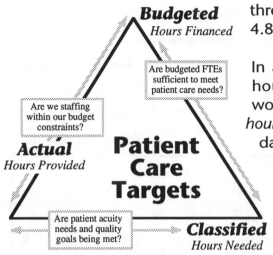

Figure 4.5 Patient Care Targets

threshold of ± 5%, the manager in Exhibit 4.8 clearly did not meet the target.

In an ideal world the *budgeted* HPM or hours of care per patient day (HPPD) would reflect the average acuity, that is, *hours needed, or classified,* on the average day. Also ideally, the manager would *actually provide* those hours. (See Figure 4.5.) In the real world, however, a crystal ball would be needed to anticipate and staff to an often unknown volume and acuity—and a magic wand to instantly create, or eliminate, staff members at a moment's notice.

Benchmarking

So... you think you're good... how do you really know? Perhaps you've got an 80% success rate. Maybe improvements have been continuous—and sustained over time for the last 10 years. So what? If performance results are still in the bottom 10% of the community sample, you're not going to be able to compete for managed care contracts and public choice. Even if the organization's prices are the lowest, managed care companies may not want to sign on or subject their patients to poorly performing services. While exaggerated to make a point, performance results must be compared—not only to their past performance—but to others who are performing similar work. And the need to compare beyond the community is now present. Ask yourself this question: If you needed a heart transplant and knew the survival rate was "X" at the local hospital, but the rate zoomed to "5X" if you got on a plane and went to Transplantville, USA, what would you do?

The above is a simple demonstration of **benchmarking,** a way of measuring and comparing organizational results to a standard of excellence. Knowing what and where best practices are occurring can help organizations in several ways. Identifying the best of the best:

- Provides an external reality check on performance results

- Sets the pace while helping others set realistic targets

- Provides a point of reference from which measured evaluations may be made

- Identifies a population of customers who can be surveyed about why they think their supplier organization is "the best"

Resource Utilization Report Card

Modality Description or Patient Class Level	Sunday	Monday	Tuesday	Wednesday	Thursday	Friday	Saturday	Sunday	Monday	Tuesday	Wednesday	Thursday	Friday	Saturday	Total Modalities or Patient Days	Hours per Modality (HPM) or Patient Day (HPPD)	Total Classified (Weighted & Acuity Required) Hours
Speech Therapy		20	10	20	10	20			20	10	20	10	20		160	1.0	160
Physical Therapy		50	50	50	50	50			50	50	50	50	50		500	1.0	500
Risk Factor Consult		20	10	20	10	20			20	10	20	10	20		160	1.5	240
Recreation Therapy		20	10	20	10	20			20	10	20	10	20		160	.5	80
Occupational Therapy		20	20	20	20	20			20	20	20	20	20		200	1.0	200
Vocational Rehab		20	10	20	10	20			20	10	20	10	20		160	1.5	240
TOTALS		150	110	150	110	150			150	110	150	110	150		1340		1420

A. Total pay period patient days or modalities _____ 1340

B. Total weighted required hours (from above) _____ 1420

C. Total hours actually provided (source: payroll, Productivity and Acuity Report, or a simple manual count of actual staffed hours). _____ 1600

D. Hours per patient day or modality:
  1) **Budget** (the standard remains constant throughout fiscal year) _____ 1.0
  2) **Classified** (weighted and acuity required) [B ÷ A] _____ 1.1
  3) **Actual** staffed hours provided [C ÷ A] _____ 1.2

E. Productivity Indexes (using figures from D.1, D.2, and D.3 for formulas)

  1) Actual staffed hours provided to budgeted hours: $\dfrac{\text{Hours Provided}}{\text{Hours Budgeted}}$ or $\dfrac{\text{D.3}}{\text{D.1}}$ _____ 120%

  2) Actual staffed hours provided to classified hours: $\dfrac{\text{Hours Provided}}{\text{Hours Required}}$ or $\dfrac{\text{D.3}}{\text{D.2}}$ _____ 109%

Exhibit 4.8 Rehabilitation Biweekly Classification Report

Resource Utilization Report Card

Modality Description or Patient Class Level	Sunday	Monday	Tuesday	Wednesday	Thursday	Friday	Saturday	Sunday	Monday	Tuesday	Wednesday	Thursday	Friday	Saturday	Total Modalities or Patient Days	Hours per Modality (HPM) or Patient Day (HPPD)	Total Classified (Weighted & Acuity Required) Hours
Classification Level #1	+	+	+	+	+	+	+	+	+	+	+	+	+	=	X	NA	=
Classification Level #2	10	5	5	0	0	0	0	0	10	10	5	0	0	0	45	3.0	135
Classification Level #3	20	20	15	15	10	0	0	10	20	10	10	10	20	20	180	4.5	810
Classification Level #4	10	20	20	25	30	30	30	25	10	20	30	30	20	10	310	6.0	1860
Classification Level #5																12.0	
Classification Level #6																24.0	
TOTALS	40	45	40	40	40	30	30	35	40	40	45	40	40	30	535		2805

A. Total pay period patient days or modalities   **535**

B. Total weighted required hours (from above)   **2805**

C. Total hours actually provided (source: payroll, Productivity and Acuity Report, or a simple manual count of actual staffed hours).   **2415**

D. Hours per patient day or modality:
1) **Budget** (the standard remains constant throughout fiscal year)   **4.0**
2) **Classified** (weighted and acuity required) [B ÷ A]   **5.2**
3) **Actual** staffed hours provided [C ÷ A]   **4.5**

E. Productivity Indexes (using figures from D.1, D.2, and D.3 for formulas)

1) Actual staffed hours provided to budgeted hours: $\dfrac{\text{Hours Provided}}{\text{Hours Budgeted}}$ or $\dfrac{D.3}{D.1}$ **113%**

2) Actual staffed hours provided to classified hours: $\dfrac{\text{Hours Provided}}{\text{Hours Required}}$ or $\dfrac{D.3}{D.2}$ **87%**

Exhibit 4.9 Patient-Care Unit Biweekly Classification Report

- Pinpoints processes to be analyzed to discover how the best results are achieved

Benchmarking is easy to practice internally. Look around in your organization. Who gives the best customer service to you... an internal customer? Who gives the best external customer service? Which departments have fewer delays, less rework, fewer complaints? Who consistently meets or exceeds their outcome, process, and cost outcomes? The more you know, the easier it is to improve. And improvement doesn't always mean starting from scratch and reinventing the wheel. Much can be learned from others' mistakes and successes by communicating and sharing performance results.

Report Cards: Sharing Data and Communicating with MCOs and Other Customers

Reporting performance results is possibly the most important communication organizations can provide to their customers—both internal and external. Healthcare organizations that have been proclaiming that they give high-quality care are now being asked—by self-insured businesses, MCOs, even the news media—to provide the data. Everyone wants to know how well, as evidenced by tangible, measurable results, things are going. The written evidence is typically referred to as a *report card*. Most of us are (all too) familiar with report cards from our school days. They sent a measurable message home to our parents about how well we were performing in different subjects at school. As students, we got information about which subjects needed more of our attention. The school board, on the other hand, looking at schools across the community, compared and analyzed report card grades and other performance results data to measure how well the teachers were teaching.

There are many other types of "report cards" that touch our lives. Movie reviews are subjective report cards from "experts" in the field, whom we may or may not respect. However, the more objective data—dollars earned—may be the report card that nudges us to go see the movie. Just as in other aspects of our lives, in the healthcare industry, report cards take on many different forms. The **Resource Utilization Report Card**, Exhibits 4.8 and 4.9 are examples of an objective, financially focused report card. Benchmarking data—previously discussed—can also be used for report cards.

When creating a report card, it's important to remember that diverse customer groups will want different information. Overloading a group with information they don't need or want is a mistake you don't want to make, so plan to have more than one report card format. When presenting data about a clinical path, for example, *MCOs, business groups,* and the *general public* will want cost and quality data. The *Board* will want the bottom line data, quality outcome, market results, and financial performance data. *Medical staff* will want information pertinent to their practice patterns. *Employees* will want to know about their contribution and the impact it made on results. Thus, report cards will take on many different forms and depths, depending on who will be receiving the information. The following pages contain examples of report cards. They're all different because they address different audiences who have different interests and uses for the information. However, each responds to a set of criteria that should be included each time a report card is generated.

Report Card Criteria
Ask the following when generating a report card:

- *Who is the audience? To whom are we accountable? Who will receive this information?*

- *Target the audience. Ask what measures are appropriate for this purpose? What information does this audience want?*

- *Compare data results over time. Are trends apparent? Is there evidence of improvement results being sustained over time?*

- *Don't forget the external customer. It's not required; however, if you don't supply it, someone else will, and it may not be correct. Ask yourself if you'd rather your customers receive the data from you, the newspaper, or an MCO?*

Several examples of report cards have been included on the following pages. The first, from Butterworth Health System in Grand Rapids, Michigan, is a **Report Card for Outcomes Management** (Exhibit 4.10). It is an ideal example of information clinical pathway teams need to help them solve problems, improve processes, and eliminate steps. The report is rich in baseline information, clinical outcome data, both internal and external comparative data, patient satisfaction survey results, and cost and utilization data—something that is too rarely seen on this type of report. This report is the future. Business will be accrued and sustained on the basis of both cost and quality outcomes. Therefore, every decision every manager and his or her natural work team or cross-functional team make must be based on the same formula: cost and quality outcomes.

Report Card for Outcomes Management
BUTTERWORTH HEALTH SYSTEM

Pathway: MYOCARDIAL INFARCTION   Date: June 96
DRG: 121 & 122

This report is prepared pursuant to but not limited to (P.A. 368 OF 1978). This report is a review function and as such is confidential and shall be used only for the purpose provided by law and shall not be a public record and shall not be available for court subpoena.

PATIENT CASE-MIX

Patient Descriptors

Avg. # MIs/month = 50
37% female, 63% male
Average age: 68
CHF at admission = 24%
% previous MI = 25%
% smoker = 40%
% AntSept MI = 34%

Patient Interventions

% of Thrombolytic = 29%
% Direct PTCA = 7%
% of Catheterization = 72%
% of PTCA = 21%
% of CABG = 16%
% with IV Heparin = 69%

CURRENT IMPROVEMENT ACTIVITIES

1. Reduce time from admit to direct angioplasty
2. Use of troponin & myoglobin
3. Better lipid monitoring by adding baseline level to ED draw
4. Expand use of SF 36 to non-cardiac rehab population
5. Decrease time to consults

OUTCOMES

Patient Satisfaction Overall quality of care question from patient satisfaction survey

	Oct-Dec/95	Jan-Mar/96
Cardiovascular	4.64	4.49
MCC	4.57	4.67

Areas for improvement
Ease of finding way around hospital
Noise level when patient needs rest

Clinical Outcomes NRMI 12/95

Symptom(s) onset to drug .... 140 min
Time to thrombolytic .... 33 min
Total stroke rate 0.5%
Recurrent ischemia 10%
Recurrent MI 3%
B Blockers at discharge (DC) 43%
ASA at DC 83%
Ca Channel Blockers at DC 32%
ACE Inhibitors at DC 22%

Functional Health Status
Cardiac rehab enrollee post MI with SF36 tool, top score of 100, N=36

	Pre-Rehab	6 Months
Mental health	71	70
Emotional role	60	89
Social function	70	65
Vitality	49	57
General health	62	73
Pain	67	70
Physical role	38	63
Physical function	62	83

Cost and Utilization DRG 122

	1995	1996 (ytd)
Length of stay	4.6	3.8
Charges/case	$7,900	$6,200
% Entering rehab	15%	25%

Exhibit 4.10 Report Card. Audience: Specific Internal Department(s)
Contributed by: Janice Schriefer, RN, MSN, MBA, CCRN, Director of Outcomes Management, Butterworth Health System, Grand Rapids, Michigan.

Quality.

It's nothing new for Baptist Health Systems

Baptist Health Systems of South Florida is happy to announce that our Dade County hospitals have earned top marks from the State of Florida.

Happy, but not surprised – because we put an emphasis on continuous quality improvement before it was a buzzword. Baptist Health Systems' physicians and employees have always been committed to the highest standards of care. And, over the years, our hospitals have received the recognition that matters most – the warm thanks of tens of thousands of patients.

The state's report analyzed length of stay, charges, and patient mortality in more than a dozen medical specialties. When Baptist Hospital, South Miami Hospital, and Homestead Hospital placed among the top 15 percent of all Florida hospitals *23* times – it was wonderful. It was also our mission.

Baptist Health Systems of South Florida. Quality care. From day one.

Baptist Health Systems of South Florida

BAPTIST HOSPITAL OF MIAMI ■ SOUTH MIAMI HOSPITAL
HOMESTEAD HOSPITAL ■ MARINERS HOSPITAL

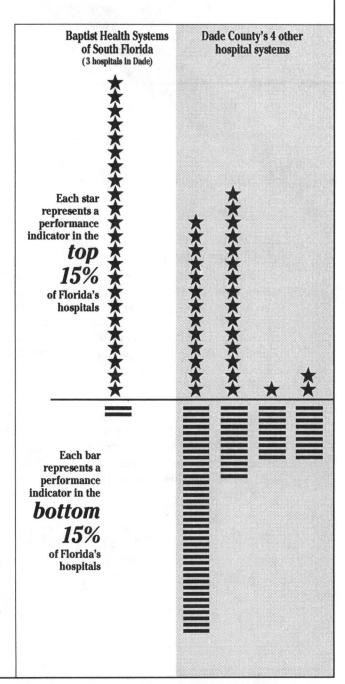

Baptist Health Systems of South Florida (3 hospitals in Dade)

Dade County's 4 other hospital systems

Each star represents a performance indicator in the *top* **15%** of Florida's hospitals

Each bar represents a performance indicator in the *bottom* **15%** of Florida's hospitals

Exhibit 4.11 Report Card. Audience: The Public, MCOs, Businesses
Contributed by: Jo Baxter, Corporate Vice President • Baptist Health Systems of South Florida, Miami, Florida.

The direction of healthcare costs at Baptist Hospital

1989
1990
1991
1992
1993
June 30, 1994

Baptist isn't waiting for healthcare reform.

While the nation has been struggling to create a new, affordable healthcare program, Baptist Hospital has been taking action. In an 18-month period (January 1993 – June 1994), Baptist reduced the average cost per admission by 5.1% over 1992.

How are we doing it? A Continuous Quality Improvement process, bench-marking, medical practice guidelines and caremapping are some of the innovative concepts used at Baptist to lower expenses while enhancing quality of care.

Baptist was also the first hospital in South Florida to install Iameter, a sophisticated computer system which tracks inpatient costs, utilization and quality. Our doctors, nurses and ancillary staff can now streamline patient care by coordinating tests and procedures, avoiding duplication and unnecessary services, and focusing on the most cost-effective drugs, supplies and therapies.

It all boils down to Baptist Hospital's Value Initiative, our strategic formula for the '90s: High Quality + Low Cost = Value. It's a simple equation, but a serious commitment.

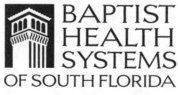

BAPTIST HEALTH SYSTEMS OF SOUTH FLORIDA

8900 North Kendall Drive • Miami, FL

Exhibit 4.12 Report Card. Audience: The Public, MCOs, Businesses
Contributed by: Jo Baxter, Corporate Vice President • Baptist Health Systems of South Florida, Miami, Florida.

Exhibits 4.11 and 4.12 are print ads for Baptist Health Systems in Miami, Florida. This organization enjoys an excellent reputation in its community and can back it up with hard data—as evidenced in these two ads. The real strength of the ads, as report cards, comes from the emphasis on cost. The message that is coming out loud and clear is that this system not only provides great care but can do so at a competitive cost. These ads are really report cards for MCOs, businesses, and the general public, who can still exert a fair amount of pressure on businesses and MCOs to respond to their needs as customers.

Exhibit 4.13, **Strategic Outcomes Report Card**, is important because everything that is pursued organizationally must link back to the mission, the vision, and the strategic priorities. If progress toward those priorities is measured and reported, it will remain a priority for the people who are responsible for the outcomes, and the outcomes will be more likely to be achieved.

The **Internal Supplier Report Card**, (Exhibit 4.14) is a report card that is growing in popularity. Most healthcare organizations have sought customer feedback from patients, physicians, and even employees. However, internal customers are often partners in care and have a huge impact on whether or not the care was successful. More and more organizations are paying close attention to the internal customer and setting expectations about behavior and coownership of outcomes. Just as the physician report card and patient satisfaction survey results affect the evaluations of a nursing unit, internal customer feedback is being included in more and more merit evaluations of support departments.

Last, Exhibit 4.15, **Communication Report Plan and Report Card**, combines planning with reporting. Created by Saint Joseph Hospital & Health Center, in Kokomo, Indiana, it serves several purposes. One, the layout forced the organization to plan—to assess who received information, whether they needed it, and how often they needed it. Two, it was in a report card format, so results could be reported out to the board, performance improvement steering committee, medical staff, or individual functions and departments. Three, it served as an ongoing source of who was getting what information. So everyone knew what everyone knew and what they didn't know.

In the years to come, we'll see more and more report cards, and they will get increasingly sophisticated and glossy. The critical factor for those of us who work in healthcare is not how polished the report is but the reliability and validity of the data. Given that, in the absence of reliable data, users will reach for whatever data are available, we can never let go of our responsibility for assessing and reporting results... no matter how we feel about statistics.

Strategic Outcomes Report Card
XYZ HEALTH SYSTEM

To: Board of Trustees   Date: March 1997

OUTCOMES

	Not Met	Met	Exceeded

Strategic Priority #1:
Fully Functional Integrated Delivery System

	Not Met	Met	Exceeded
• Merge or joint venture with facilities sharing our mission and values.	☐	☒	☐
• Expand ambulatory services throughout the organization, to support every clinical path.	☐	☐	☒
• Bring home health care services into the continuum of care.	☐	☒	☐
• Bring key physicians on-line with hospital-based information systems.	☒	☐	☐

Strategic Priority #2:
A Provider of Safe, Cost-effective Care

	Not Met	Met	Exceeded
• Cost per discharge ± 2% of target	☐	☒	☐
• Safety statistics (employees, patients, etc.)	☐	☒	☐
• Cost per ambulatory surgery	☐	☒	☐

Strategic Priority #3:
Improve patient clinical and satisfaction outcomes

	Not Met	Met	Exceeded
• Achieve overall patient satisfaction rating 4.5.	☐	☐	☒
• Reduce unscheduled returns to OR and ICU.	☐	☒	☐
• Enroll all smokers in cessation program.	☒	☐	☐
• Expand use of cardiac rehab program to all cardiac patients.	☒	☐	☐

Exhibit 4.13 Report Card. Audience: Board of Directors, Medical Staff, All Managers, and Employees

Internal Supplier Report Card

Contacts:	**Courtesy/Effectiveness**	**Comments and suggestions are encouraged.**
N = None	Not met = 0	However, if your expectations, as a customer, are "not
O = Occasional	Met = 1	met," comments are required. State expectations,
R = Routine	Exceeded = 2	desired outcomes, or specific improvement ideas.
K = Key Supplier		

Contacts   *Courtesy*   *Effectiveness*

Supplier/Function	Contacts	Courtesy	Effectiveness	Customer/Function __Critical Care__
Admitting	R	1	O	A contingency plan is needed for a more efficient transfer of patients on 3-11/11-7.
EKG/EEG	R	2	2	
Endoscopy Center	O	1	1	
Pharmacy IV Therapy	K	2	2	
Radiation	O	1	2	
Dialysis	O	1	1	
Materials Mgmt. Central Service	R	2	O	Supplies are coming to the floor without stickers making it difficult to hold staff accountable for charging.
Materials Mgmt. Mail Room	N	O	O	
Materials Mgmt. Linen Room	R	2	1	Deliver linens in the evening. Then beds could be changed at the patient's convenience.
Materials Mgmt. Purchasing	O	1	1	

Exhibit 4.14 Report Card. Audience: Senior and Mid-Level Managers

Saint Joseph Hospital & Health Center
Risk, Quality, and Utilization Management Report

August 1996

Department/Team Reports	Times/year reported				Significant Issues (+ or −), identified during the quarter	Summary of findings and actions
	Department or Function	Steering/PI Committee	Board/Senior Management	Medical Staff		
Medical Staff Departments/Services						
Anesthesia	VR*	VR*	4	4	*VR Variance Report	
Emergency	VR	VR	4	4		
Surgery	VR	VR	4	4		
Medicine	VR	VR	4	4		
Radiology	VR	VR	4	4		
Nuclear cardiology	VR	VR	4	4		
Radiation oncology	VR	VR	4	4		
Psychiatry	VR	VR	4	4		
Respiratory	VR	VR	4	4		
OB/GYN	VR	VR	4	4		
Pathology	VR	VR	2	2		
Review Functions						
Infection control	VR	VR	4	4		
Drug utilization	VR	VR	AR**	AR**	**AR As Received	
Surgical case review	VR	VR	4	4		
Blood utilization	VR	VR	4	4		
Medical records	VR	VR	4	4		
Utilization review	VR	VR	4	4		
Primary Operating Objectives Teams						
• Clinical pathways	Ongoing	12 Updates	6	12 Updates	Clinical pathways for chest pain, normal vaginal deliveries, C/S, and normal newborn will be inserviced with nursing staff this month and implemented the first week in September.	The team has identified the next group of care maps to be completed. Recommendations from the Critical Care Committee were used in helping to determine the next DRGs on which to focus the committee's efforts.
• Patient Care Redesign	Ongoing	12 Updates	6	12 Updates	The steering team received reports from the subcommittee leaders and a new timetable was approved for proceeding with implementation of the 4th floor and the expanded care team.	Due to JCAHO survey and the timing of education, the original implementation date in early December had to be delayed. The steering team concurred with the Enlarging the Care Team recommendation for timing of implementation of their next phase. Care Management Team completed their work and the pilot program has now become a fully operational program.
Cross-Functional Teams						
• ER Team	Ongoing	12 Updates	6	12 Updates	The original ER team completed its recommendations which were made to an ad hoc committee to expedite changes in the ER.	Plans are being completed to redesign the Triage area, develop protocols for nursing to facilitate movement of patients through the system and development and implementation of a patient satisfaction survey.

Exhibit 4.15 Communication Report Plan and Report Card. Audience: Board of Directors *(Continues)*
Contributed by: Polly A. Jones, CCSW, Director Quality & Resource Management • Saint Joseph Hospital & Health Center, Kokomo, Indiana.

Saint Joseph Hospital & Health Center
Risk, Quality, and Utilization Management Report

August 1996

Department/ Team Reports	Times/year reported				Significant Issues (+ or –), identified during the quarter	Summary of findings and actions
	Department or Function	Steering/PI Committee	Board/Senior Management	Medical Staff		
Cross-Functional Teams (con't)						
• Medical Records Team	Ongoing	12 Updates	6	4	Team initiated to meet JCAHO requirements for multidisciplinary Medical Records Team that meets quarterly. Team met in June.	Already reported.
• Duplicate Medical Records Team	Ongoing	12 Updates	6	12 Updates	Team has gathered data at a determined rate of occurrence and has gathered and reviewed forms to determine all places information is entered. Looking at common elements and changing forms to ensure information is being asked for and entered in the same way.	Now researching capabilities of computer to determine ability to search for someone in more than one format, e.g., name, social security number, birthdate, to determine if person is already in the system under a different name. Or, is there a glitch in the system?
Natural Work Teams						
• CP Lab Team	Ongoing	12 Updates	6	12 Updates	Need to redesign processes to accommodate problems with scheduling and reading of tests.	Time study completed on the wait times relate to transporting patients to and from the department. Data being tabulated for review by team.
• Food Services Team	Ongoing	12 Updates	6	12 Updates	Food Services natural work team is being reinstituted to continue work on redesigning processes.	To begin meeting in August.
Volume, Casemix, Utilization Indicators	12	VR	4	4		
Top 10 DRGs	4	4	4	4		
DCNHS or "System" Clinical Indicators					For all clinical indicators, report benchmark data comparing performance results to:	
• Readmission rate	4	4	4	4	• Your own past performance	
• Unsched. readmit rate	4	4	4	4	• Others in your system	
• Amb. surg. unsched. admit	4	4	4	4	• National database statistics	
• Unsched. return to ICU	4	4	4	4		
• Neonatal mortality	4	4	4	4		
• Primary C-sections	4	4	4	4		
• Repeat C-sections	4	4	4	4		
• Overall C-sections	4	4	4	4		
• Successful VBAC	4	4	4	4		
• Incomplete MR rate	4	4	4	4		
• Surgical wound infection	4	4	4	4		
• Unsched. return to OR	4	4	4	4		
• Perioperative mortality	4	4	4	4		
• Falls resulting in injury	4	4	4	4		

Exhibit 4.15 Continued

(Continues)

Saint Joseph Hospital & Health Center
Risk, Quality, and Utilization Management Report

August 1996

Department/ Team Reports	Times/year reported				Significant Issues (+ or –), identified during the quarter	Summary of findings and actions
	Department or Function	Steering/PI Committee	Board/Senior Management	Medical Staff		
Worker Compensation and Loss	Per Incident	0	4	0		
Safety Activity Report	0	0	6	0		
Claims and Litigation	0	0	6	0		
Medication Errors	0	0	4	4		
Patient Care Provider Report	0	0	4	4		
Patient Satisfaction	4	4	4	4		

Reporting to the Governing Board
Issues Saint Joseph's Considered

Reasons for reporting
- Ultimate responsibility for the organization rests with the Board
- Strategic planning
- JCAHO requirement
- Oversight requirement if part of a larger healthcare system
- Advertise/communicate successes—Identify opportunities for improvement
- Identify trends/problems which need intervention at the Board level

What to report
- QI activities hospital and medical staff
    - Team reports
    - External comparative reports benchmarking
- On-going monitors, e.g., blood utilization, infection control, surgical case review
- Utilization Experience
    - Casemix
    - Denials
    - LOS Top 10 DRGs
    - Units of service from ancillary departments
- Risk Management
    - Potential and actual claims
    - Safety Committee Activities
    - Workers' Compensation employee incidents, injuries, lost days
    - Litigation Update
    - Incident reports patients and visitors

Components and Format
- Matrix model works best.
- Include benchmarking data where available both internal and external, e.g., mortality rates compared to peer hospitals or the state/national rates for a specific DRG.
- Use comparison data for internal statistical reports, e.g., infection rates for current quarter vs. previous quarter.
- Quantify data e.g., 95% of patients met standards versus 19 patients met standards.
- Identify actions in place or being developed for opportunities for improvement.

Frequency
This will vary by organization. A minimum of quarterly is recommended to ensure timeliness of information, continuous reminders of performance improvement activities, and to promote on-going feedback and recommendations from Board. Stagger reports so the Board is not overwhelmed with data.

Exhibit 4.15 Continued

Notes

1. W.E. Deming, *Out of Crisis* (Cambridge, MA: Center for Advanced Engineering Study, Massachusetts Institute of Technology, 1986).

2. K. Bernowski, "The Quality Glossary," *Quality Progress* (February 1992): 25.

Recommended Reading

Can variance tracking avert potential risk management disaster? 1995. *Hospital Case Management.* December: 181–183.

Don't let wound care scar your case management program. 1996. *Hospital Case Management.* March: 33–35.

Line-item data help hospital improve, win managed care contracts. 1996. *QI/TQM.* March: 25–28.

Quality data give hospitals the edge in MCO contracting. 1995. *Hospital Peer Review.* December: 170–173.

The report card season is now here: Will your hospital make the grade? 1994. *Hospital Peer Review.* December: 181–184.

Alba, T. et al. 1994. How hospitals can use internal benchmark data to create effective managed care arrangements. *Managed Care Quarterly.* Spring: 79–89.

Alsever, R. 1995. Developing a hospital report card to demonstrate value in healthcare. *Journal for Healthcare Quality.* January–February: 19–28.

DeToro, I. 1995. The 10 pitfalls of Benchmarking. *Quality Progress.* January: 61–63.

Kennedy, M. 1994. Applying benchmarking to the clinical arena. *The Quality Letter for Healthcare Leaders.* November: 2–10.

Laffel, G. 1995. Developing a corporate-level performance assessment system. *Quality Management in Health Care.* Summer: 62–70.

Lambertus, T. 1995. Strategies for leaping major obstacles in benchmarking. *Hospital Benchmarks.* April: 47–49.

Montet, L. 1994. From the cutting edge—tips on developing hospital report cards. *MPR Exchange.* November–December: 2–3.

Myers, D. and Heller, J. 1995. The dual role of AT&T's self-assessment process. *Quality Progress.* January: 79–83.

Spath, P. 1994. Choose quality indicators wisely in preparing for your report card. *Hospital Peer Review.* September: 144–148.

Taylor, G., and Morgan, M. 1995. The reverse appraisal: A tool for leadership development. *Quality Progress.* December: 81–87.

White, R., and Lyons, J. 1994. "Road maps" more practical now than "report cards." *Modern Healthcare.* November 7: 56–58.

Wilson, E. 1996. Getting the FAccts straight. *Hospital Peer Review.* November-December: 12–14, 18.

IF YOU THINK
YOU'RE TOO SMALL
TO IMPROVE
PERFORMANCE RESULTS,
YOU'RE JUST NOT
THINKING
BIG ENOUGH

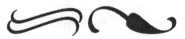

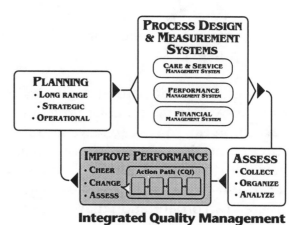

Integrated Quality Management

5. PERFORMANCE IMPROVEMENT

How's it going?

Performance improvement. It's at the core of every topic in this book. People in healthcare organizations plan, design, measure, and assess, all for the purpose of continually improving performance results. It's a worthy goal, considering the industry in which we've chosen to work. For this reason, we constantly question. What has been accomplished? What are the outcomes? What progress has been made? What impact has occurred?

The answers to these questions determine if outcomes, process, and costs meet, don't meet, or exceed the expectation, goal, or target. It is at this point that a determination for future work can be made. Is it time to problem solve, attack recurring problems, and look for broken processes to repair? Is it time to celebrate accomplishments or improvements? Or is it time to look for still more opportunities, to push to become the best of the best, a center of excellence? All of these options will be discussed in this chapter.

Scientific Method versus Inspection

For many years, organizations believed that if they inspected enough, surely a desired level of quality would be achieved. Reference the stickers that fall out of new underwear that say, "Inspected by worker #72." Quality assurance was popular in hospitals and required by accrediting agencies. But one of the most significant lessons learned from Japanese success stories is that inspections, and the crisis management style problem-solving activities that follow, do not necessarily produce quality outcomes, and even when they do, the improvements are not always sustained over time. While some inspection is necessary, if it's being used in an attempt to maintain quality, it's being misused and becomes an avoidable cost of quality—waste. Performance improvement builds on the belief that quality can be built into systems by internal experts, the people who process the workload and work with patients, families, physicians, and managed care organizations (MCOs) every day. Their involvement, from planning though performance and evaluation, is the best way to ensure predictable, high-quality results in both the superiority of the service (or product) and in the efficiency and effectiveness of the process.

We see and participate in examples of this theory every day. Some of us drive to work at a particular time every day, following a route we know we can count on, so we can leave at the last possible moment and still make it to work on time. Others choose to leave a half an hour earlier, because in addition to on-time arrival they also want a stress-free, relaxing drive to work, which can only be achieved at an earlier hour. Once at work, most of us are in an organization that is using an electronic device that guarantees a phone will be answered within two to three rings. Knowing that most customers prefer a "live" voice, the robot will first give human operators an opportunity to answer, but if the operators are busy, the electronic device will dutifully pick up, within the acceptable number of rings.

So the question becomes, how are these systems developed, and how is quality built into them? The answer is a scientific method—the process of improving performance.

Performance Improvement Action Path

If you want to improve performance results—and sustain the results over time—you have to change the process or the system (group of processes). The scientific method displayed in Figure 5.1, **Performance Improvement Action Path,** is one process that can be used to change and improve other processes. Physicians use this scientific method all the time as they study our individual health problems. For example, when most people go to their physician, they present a list of symptoms: "I have pain in my shoulder, my arm itches so much it's keeping me up all night, and I have a headache." As the patient runs down the list of maladies, the physician is listening, questioning, and running a list of *possible problems* through his or her mental computer, keeping some as possibilities and rejecting others. The physician is in the *Project Selection* phase, and the goal is to narrow the issue so he or she can resolve it. Sometimes, there are several illnesses occurring at the same time, which complicate this part of the process.

As the physician gathers more information about the issue, and it becomes more focused, his or her attention turns to what might be *causing* the problem—*Cause Analysis & Evidence*—the root cause. Sometimes, in medicine, the root cause is unknown, and physicians are forced to treat the symptoms, as in the case of arthritis. However, even when that is the case, they still pursue data to verify the root cause, because a diagnosis of arthritis, in itself, gives physicians information useful to improving the situation, even when a cure cannot be achieved. They zero in on the assumed root cause

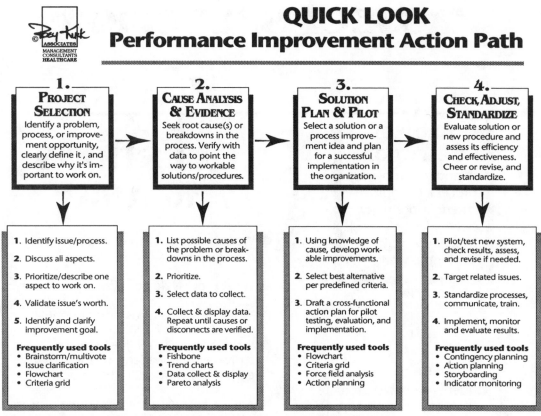

QUICK LOOK
Performance Improvement Action Path

1. PROJECT SELECTION	2. CAUSE ANALYSIS & EVIDENCE	3. SOLUTION PLAN & PILOT	4. CHECK, ADJUST, STANDARDIZE
Identify a problem, process, or improvement opportunity, clearly define it, and describe why it's important to work on.	Seek root cause(s) or breakdowns in the process. Verify with data to point the way to workable solutions/procedures.	Select a solution or a process improvement idea and plan for a successful implementation in the organization.	Evaluate solution or new procedure and assess its efficiency and effectiveness. Cheer or revise, and standardize.
1. Identify issue/process. 2. Discuss all aspects. 3. Prioritize/describe one aspect to work on. 4. Validate issue's worth. 5. Identify and clarify improvement goal. **Frequently used tools** • Brainstorm/multivote • Issue clarification • Flowchart • Criteria grid	1. List possible causes of the problem or breakdowns in the process. 2. Prioritize. 3. Select data to collect. 4. Collect & display data. Repeat until causes or disconnects are verified. **Frequently used tools** • Fishbone • Trend charts • Data collect & display • Pareto analysis	1. Using knowledge of cause, develop workable improvements. 2. Select best alternative per predefined criteria. 3. Draft a cross-functional action plan for pilot testing, evaluation, and implementation. **Frequently used tools** • Flowchart • Criteria grid • Force field analysis • Action planning	1. Pilot/test new system, check results, assess, and revise if needed. 2. Target related issues. 3. Standardize processes, communicate, train. 4. Implement, monitor and evaluate results. **Frequently used tools** • Contingency planning • Action planning • Storyboarding • Indicator monitoring

Figure 5.1 Performance Improvement Action Path

by collecting data—for example, lab tests and radiology studies—in order to confirm assumptions with hard data. Once the assumptions are confirmed—or challenged and changed—by the data, a "real" root cause is revealed. It's easy for most of us to see how the real root cause of a medical problem is a key to the solution, or cure. If a bacterial infection is the root cause, take antibiotics; if an appendix is rupturing, surgery may be the only resolution.

If the real root cause has been verified, the third phase of the scientific method, **Solution Plan & Pilot**, is pretty straightforward. Once there are data to confirm a diagnosis, there are time-tested medical protocols that guide physicians in their treatment determination. However, today's physicians must weigh the solution they recommend on factors besides whether or not it will resolve the medical problem. One big issue is whether or not the MCO will reimburse for the treatment. Another is support for patients after the treatment: do they live alone, can they manage by themselves, is transportation a problem—just to name a few. Thus, planning for a successful implementation of the treatment regime is essential to a successful outcome.

How does one know if there's been a successful outcome? In the case of a medical situation, it's pretty easy to ascertain. The pain goes away. The itch

PROJECT SELECTION

1.
PROJECT SELECTION
Identify a problem, process, or improvement opportunity, clearly define it , and describe why it's important to work on.

1. Identify a broad issue, process, or procedure.

2. Brainstorm and discuss all aspects.

3. Prioritize, select, and clarify one aspect to pursue.

4. Project time needed to improve and agree that the possible return is worth the time spent.

5. Identify and clarify improvement goal.

QUESTIONS TO ASK

- What is the problem or issue you want to resolve?

- What process do you want to improve?

- Which aspect is a customer priority?

- Is there a gap in service between customer (i.e., patient, physician, employee) expectations and delivery?

- Are we following the prescribed process on a routine basis?

- Are the results what we expected? Are they reliable and predictable?

- Is this the core issue or is it a complex problem?

TOOLS TO USE

RECOMMENDED TOOLS
Brainstorming & Multivoting
Flowchart · Criteria Grid
Cost-Benefit Analysis
Issue Clarification

OTHER USEFUL TOOLS
Fishbone (Cause & Effect) Diagram
Trend (Run) Chart · Pareto Analysis
Data Collection & Data Display Tools
Action Planning & Recording
Indicator Monitoring

stops itching. The leg can bear weight. The heart starts beating. The patient can return to normal activities. These are indicators that can be used for the last phase of the scientific method: **Check, Adjust, Standardize**. Once again, upon checking, the indicator will be met, not met, or exceeded. If it's not met, adjustments can be made to the treatment plan. Once the indicator is met on an ongoing basis, the process can be standardized; become standard operating procedure; and go into the procedure manual for communication, education, and reference purposes.

Project Selection: Case Study Phase 1

Switching from the medical example, we'll apply the scientific method to a management of care problem that occurred at a community hospital. The organization had just begun implementing a formal process for improving organizational performance. One of the biggest obstacles to a successful implementation was the medical staff who ~~resisted~~ refused to participate in the process. Acknowledging that the physicians were very important customers, the Quality Council was reluctant to move forward without their involvement. After much discussion, they decided to involve the physicians as customers, hoping that if they solved some issues for the physicians, perhaps they would be more agreeable to participating in the future. They surveyed the physicians to identify which organizational processes were causing them, or their staff, the most frustration, time, or dollars.

Consensus was reached quickly that the waiting time for outpatient procedures was the issue that was most frustrating to everyone. Subsequently, a team consisting of representatives from all of the departments offering outpatient services was charged with resolving the issue. First, they looked at what was happening. Patients were waiting up to 2 hours to register for their procedures. They were complaining to the physicians' offices. Registration clerks were overloaded and being identified as the root cause of the problem—even before the problem was defined. Physicians were threatening to refer their patients elsewhere. As with most young teams, every time the group identified something that was wrong, someone (or some department) was blamed, and everyone rushed to solution. They even reached a quick consensus that it was the registration clerks who were at fault, and if salaries could be increased so that better caliber people could be hired, that would certainly solve the problem! Holding them back to study the problem and find the real root cause was a constant challenge.

Finally, however, they did agree that they would work on the issue of delays in outpatient registration. After talking with patients and physicians, they set a goal to have patients wait no longer than 5 minutes. The team asked for 3 months to study and resolve the issue and did a cost-benefit analysis to

CAUSE ANALYSIS & EVIDENCE

2.
CAUSE ANALYSIS & EVIDENCE

Seek root cause(s) or breakdowns in the process. Verify with data to point the way to workable solutions/procedures.

1. List possible causes of the problem or break-downs in the process.

2. Prioritize "perceived" causes of the problem or process disconnects.

3. Select data to collect that will support, rule out, or validate cause of failure.

4. Collect and display data. Repeat until all causes or disconnects are verified and con-census is reached.

QUESTIONS TO ASK

■ What are the *possible* root causes? Why is this occurring? Is the process not working, or are we not following a good process?

■ Of the *possible* root causes, which show promise to be the *real* root cause?

■ What data will verify that our possible root cause is a reality?*

■ What is the best way to collect it?

■ What does the data say?

■ Are we able to back up or substantiate the *possible* root cause with hard data?

* All *possible* root causes must be verified. Otherwise, they are only assumptions. If you create and implement a solution based on an incorrect assumption, it won't improve the process or the subsequent outcome.

TOOLS TO USE

RECOMMENDED TOOLS

Fishbone Diagram
Trend Charts
Data Collection Tools · Task List
Data Display Tools
Pareto Analysis

OTHER USEFUL TOOLS

Brainstorming & Multivoting
Flowchart
Action Planning & Recording

show the potential return on investment and justify the cost of the team. The Quality Council approved the project, and asked the team to check in at the end of each phase of the scientific method, and they began their quest.

Cause Analysis & Evidence: Case Study Phase 2

Once the project was approved, the team jumped (both feet) into the blame game. Everyone had an opinion about who, or what department, was at fault. As stated previously, most members of the team believed that the breakdown was somewhere in the registration process because that is where the delay occurred, so the team leader tried to get the group to flowchart the registration process. There was absolutely no consensus. Fortunately, they were rescued from their debate by one team member who pulled an approved, documented procedure, in the form of a flowchart, out of the procedure manual. Even though it was dusty, team members remembered the procedure, and some of them had followed it… for a while. At the end of the meeting, the team leader made them place their hand on the manual and vow to follow the procedure for 2 weeks while data were collected. (See Figure 5.2.)

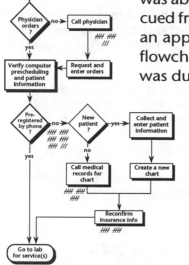

Figure 5.2 Flowchart of Outpatient Registration Process

Almost immediately, everything looked different. As departments followed the process, they not only found it useful, but they also were able to identify bottlenecks, breakdowns, and disconnects in the process. Physician orders and preregistration by phone were identified by team members as the most troublesome, but the team felt helpless because they couldn't force physicians to call with the correct orders. Also, when they asked, "Why weren't patients preregistered?" The answer almost always came back, *"We didn't know they were coming."* It became clearer and clearer that the root cause of the problem was the *customer*—the physicians—the very people the team was trying to win over. Further study of Pareto charts (Figure 5.3) showed that more than 80% of their outpatients were "walk-ins," and an even greater percentage knew about the procedure more than 24 hours

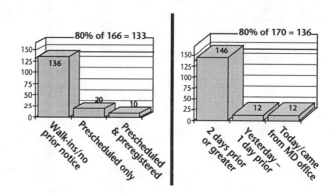

Figure 5.3 Pareto Charts of Outpatient Service Delays

SOLUTION PLAN & PILOT

3.

SOLUTION PLAN & PILOT

Select a solution or a process improvement idea and plan for a successful implementation in the organization.

1. Use knowledge of root cause or identified process failure to develop or brainstorm workable solutions and improvements.

2. Select the best realistic alternative based on predefined criteria.

3. Using representatives from all involved departments, create a cross-functional action plan for pilot testing, evaluation, and implementation.

QUESTIONS TO ASK

■ Considering the real root cause of the problem (or breakdown, bottleneck, or disconnect in the process), what are the possible solutions?

■ Which solution is the best solution? What criteria would help us prioritize and select the best solution?

■ Which has the best cost-to-benefit ratio?

■ Does one solution have fewer obstacles to a successful implementation?

■ How will we pilot and test the solution?

■ Are there people who have not been involved who should be involved in the implementation? Who will follow up?

TOOLS TO USE

RECOMMENDED TOOLS

Flowchart · Criteria Grid
Cost-Benefit Analysis
Force Field Analysis · Success Plan
Action Planning & Recording
Indicator Monitoring

OTHER USEFUL TOOLS

Brainstorming & Multivoting
Storyboarding
Action Minutes

before it was (not) scheduled to occur (Figure 5.3). It was at this point that the team started to see the possibilities ahead and believe a solution was feasible.

Solution Plan & Pilot: Case Study Phase 3

Even though the team members had learned several tools that were designed to help them come up with creative solutions, they found, in this case, that knowing the real root cause of the problem was the key to the solution. Some of their action planning is shown in Exhibit 5.1. They showed the physicians their data and at the same time pledged that if the physicians would let them know patients were coming, they would guarantee *no waiting time.* In addition, they offered to bring the physician's office staff over for a luncheon and orientation to the new notification system—which was, in essence, no more than a simple phone call. Nonetheless, they acknowledged the physician's staff as customers and armed them with a little guidebook, a phone number to call for help, and stickers for their phones with information they needed to preschedule their patients.

The new process was an immediate success, as evidenced by the huge increase in the number of patients that were able to be preregistered the day before their scheduled procedure. However, some physicians did not coop-

Action Planning Documentation

Objective What are the expected results?	Action How will results be accomplished? Specifically, what steps will be taken?	Resources needed & their cost (Labor, supplies, equipment)	Indicator How will results be measured?	• Completion Date (When) • Responsible Person (Who)
A data collection form for monitoring outpatient waiting times	• List different steps/actions related to scheduling, preregistering, and accomplishing outpatient procedures. • Create a written survey and try it out. • Teach registration clerks how to use the form to document patient waiting times to identify the bottleneck.	• 3 hours meeting time with 3–4 team members for survey development • 1 hour meeting time to train 4 registration clerks	Indicator: Areas of waiting time exceeding an acceptable range will be identified and then analyzed for resolution.	•**When:** July 1 •**Who:** Outpatient department managers, registration clerks, and team members Jeff & Jessica
Written log of registration clerk workload	• Registration clerks will log workload activities and the actual time required to accomplish tasks (time period: 2 weeks). • Team will analyze data and take action.	• Activity logs • 20 minutes documentation time daily	Indicator: Prioritized list of registration activities/tasks and required hours of workload	•**When:** July 1 •**Who:** Registration clerks
Written update of team activity for: - **Mgmt. Council** - **Quality Council** - **Steering Group**	• Team members log targeted results and action steps in meeting minutes. • Communicate progress to management council and the hospitalwide quality assessment and improvement team.	• Team meeting minutes • Secretarial hours to produce and distribute written report • Team member representation at meetings as needed	Indicator: An update will be given on team activities each Friday in the bulletin.	•**When:** Weekly •**Who:** Team members, news staff, and print shop personnel

Progress report delivered and feedback received from peers and management after each team meeting	• Post progress report of meeting on unit bulletin board.
	• Gather specific feedback to bring back to the next team meeting: acceptance, recommended revisions, suggestions for "next steps."
	  - Review at monthly unit staff meeting.
	  - Meet with unit manager individually.
		• 1 hour for staff meeting
		• 1 hour for meeting with manager
			Indicator: Employees actively participate in performance improvement process by listing recommendations or initialing acceptance of proposed changes.	•**When:** Next team meeting (ongoing)
				•**Who:** All team members

Exhibit 5.1 Outpatient Service Delays: Action Plan

CHECK, ADJUST STANDARDIZE

4.

CHECK, ADJUST, STANDARDIZE

Evaluate solution or new procedure and assess its efficiency and effectiveness. Cheer or revise, and standardize.

1. Pilot/test new system, check results, assess.

2. Tweak or make revisions if needed.

3. Target related (sub-issues or flows) or new issues to address.

4. Standardize processes, communicate details to all involved (directly or indirectly), train.

5. Implement, monitor, and evaluate results ongoing.

QUESTIONS TO ASK

■ Are the results what we expected? Are they reliable and predictable?

■ Are results meeting outcome, process, and time/cost indicators?

■ Are there any changes we should make before we make this new process a standard operating procedure?

■ How will we implement?

■ Are there people who have not been involved who should be involved in the implementation? Who will follow up?

■ Do we want to change any of the measures or measuring processes?

TOOLS TO USE

RECOMMENDED TOOLS

Data Collection Tools
Trend Charts · Success Plan
Action Planning & Recording
Storyboarding
Indicator Monitoring

OTHER USEFUL TOOLS

Brainstorming & Multivoting
Flowchart
Force Field Analysis

erate at first. When their patients, or any patients, walked in, one question was always asked, "When did you know you were coming?" If the answer was 24 hours prior, or greater, the registration clerk gave them a card with their name and phone number and said, "The next time your physician tells you to come over, call us right away. We'll call him for your orders and you won't have to wait."

Check, Adjust, Standardize: Case Study Phase 4

Checking results showed immediate improvement. For one thing, waiting time was down to almost nothing. Even the walk-ins waited less time because there was no one else waiting when they arrived. Thus, the goal that was set at the beginning of the project was successfully achieved, but that wasn't the only return on the team's investment. Outpatient Services was now a high-performing team. They were connected and work flowed easily from one department to another. They had studied, redesigned, and standardized several processes that led to improved performance results, not just in waiting time—the original mission—but in clinical and financial outcomes as well.

For example, when a physician office called to schedule lab and radiology for the same patient, all parties involved in the process knew to schedule radiology procedures first and then laboratory because the lab was better equipped to be responsive, even if a patient was delayed by the previous procedure. Another example was the guidebook that gave patient information about the test and instructions about what to do the night before. Physician offices could copy the information and give it to the patient with their own information and instructions. When registration clerks preregistered patients the night before the procedure, they asked if the patient received the information, and, if not, they would either fax it to them or read it over the phone. Also, if they knew a physician had standing protocols, and the patient did not receive them, they notified the physician's office.

The new and improved processes reduced cancellations and rework significantly. Patient satisfaction and the volume of services delivered increased at the same time the costs to deliver the services decreased. Knowing the actual costs of their services enabled them to make better decisions about which managed care contracts were profitable for the organization. All the way around, this attempt at winning over a customer paid off, in terms of quality, productivity, and financial success.

When outcomes are met, not met, or exceeded

One of the benefits of the assessment or evaluation process is the ability to learn how well, or how poorly, a natural work team or cross-functional team is performing: how close they are to target. With the help of the right indicators, comparing actual performance results to the target enables a quick, accurate assessment—the indicators are either not met, met, or exceeded. This type of assessment system is objective. No one has to figure out the meaning of "good," "average," or worst of all, "below average." Instead, energy and talent can be devoted to discovering why the indicator was met, not met, or exceeded and how to improve performance results further.

When outcomes are not met, it's usually because of one of two factors: (1) there's something wrong with the process, or (2) the process is functioning, but it's not being followed. This concept was discussed at length in Chapter 2, but it's worth repeating here as a reminder: Check to see if people are following the process, and, if they are, then review the process itself for reliability and validity. Additional ideas for what to do after performance results are analyzed in Exhibit 5.2.

Responding to managed care, competition, and capitation: What to do when costs are greater than reimbursement

Of the three possible variables, only two can be manipulated in a managed care environment because the decision to increase reimbursement is no longer an option. Organizations can change their outcomes; take a "we can't afford to do that anymore" approach; or set more realistic, achievable goals, given the available budget. Of course, administrations are very reluctant to take this position because of the fierce competition that exists and the standard of excellence they earnestly desire to achieve—and are accustomed to achieving for their patients and other customers.

Thus, if organizations can't change the reimbursement and don't want to change the expectations, that leaves only one other option—the process. They will simply have *to find a way to achieve their desired outcomes without compromising quality and without going over budget. That means streamlining the process, which means less steps.* Therefore, something needs to be left out. It might as well be something insignificant, something redundant, something that does not contribute positively toward the achievement of outcomes. It must be planned in advance in order to use the knowledge of subject matter experts and give staff members permission to let it go. Process improvement—a scientific, objective , fact-based approach—is the best path to improving quality, productivity, and cost savings concurrently. Even when teams focus *only* on improving quality outcomes, the improved process is usually more efficient and more cost effective. And that's the goal.

Communication and Planning

All performance results don't need to be reported, but it's a terrific way to

What to do when indicators are...

	Outcome	*Process*	*Time or Cost*
Not Met	• Check: Is the process being followed? • Check: Is the process viable? • Document baseline information. • Problem solve. • Check: Is the target realistic? • Prioritize.	• Identify breakdowns, bottlenecks, and disconnects in the process. • Educate staff on the new process. • Maintain the pressure until the new process or system is comfortable. • Prioritize.	• Problem solve. • Look at possible steps to eliminate or streamline. • Educate staff on the new process. • Maintain the pressure until the new process or system is comfortable.
Met	• Celebrate. • Document. • Measure other outcomes to identify other improvement opportunities. • Benchmark.	• Celebrate. • Document. • Look at other processes for improvement opportunities. • Benchmark.	• Celebrate. • Document. • Research future cost trends to anticipate and work toward future targets. • Benchmark.
Exceeded	• Celebrate and reward/recognize. • Document. • Simplify results. • Share with purchasers. • Communicate and advertise.	• Celebrate and reward/recognize. • Document. • Make it a standard operating procedure. • Share with other departments.	• Celebrate and reward/recognize. • Document. • Simplify results. • Share with purchasers. • Communicate and advertise.

Exhibit 5.2 Indicator Follow up

manage the volume of activities and hold everyone accountable for their share of the results. As stated in the beginning of the book, communication can make the difference in creating a success story. It's important to communicate throughout the process—with internal customers, patients, MCOs, physicians, and especially during implementation and follow-up activities. The reason is C-H-A-N-G-E. At best, most people are reluctant to change. As soon as the pressure is off, they will gravitate back to the comfort zone of whatever they've always done. Successful change is facilitated with participative planning and communication, so everyone knows what is expected—in both performance and results. Exhibit 5.3, **Progress Communication and Planning**, summarizes organizational measures and priorities. This provides an efficient but comprehensive look at the organizational plan for achieving the mission and vision.

Getting Started

For some, it will be challenging to start with so many other things ongoing. Most managers today are suffering from "FPS" (full-plate syndrome). If you're one of them, know that you are not alone. The only way FPS is going to get better is if *you* make it better. Prioritizing and elimination of unnecessary, noncontributing work is the only answer. Even though the "Got-a-problem-got-a-solution" method of managing has been rewarded, even idolized, it also has created and sustained many problems. Crisis management, putting out fires, and implementing quick-fix solutions will never work. They only eat up a manager's time, and their personal life, too. The easiest place to start is with your Personal Work Log Analysis, from Chapter 2. If your time is spent on the wrong things, stop. If your processes are inefficient or ineffective, study them and make changes. And under your breath, just keep saying the words *prioritize... eliminate... prioritize... eliminate...*

Healthcare managers and their staff members can't do everything for everybody anymore. However, we can prioritize what is most important to the patient's care and then ensure targeted performance results through planning, design, measurement, assessment, and ongoing performance improvement. Quality can be maintained and even maximized in a managed care environment.

Exhibit 5.3 is a matrix cross-referencing performance **MEASURES** (rows) against Strategic Priorities, P.I. Priorities, Important Functions, Dimensions of Performance, and status columns. Column abbreviations: **IDS** = Integrated Delivery System; **SCE** = Save Cost-Effective Care; **ClinO** = Clinical Outcomes; **PS-S** = Patient Satisfaction (Strategic); **PatSat** = Patient Satisfaction (P.I.); **CostEff** = Cost-Effective; **PatOut** = Patient Outcomes; **OutS** = 1. Outpatient Services; **EmD** = 2. Emergency Department; **HHC** = 3. Home Health Care; **OH** = 4. Open Heart/MI; **CritC** = 5. Critical Care; **PRgt** = Patient Rights; **PAss** = Patient Assessment; **CarePt** = Care of the Patient; **PFEd** = Patient and Family Education; **ContC** = Continuum of Care; **Lead** = Leadership; **EnvC** = Environment of Care; **HR** = Human Resources; **InfoM** = Information Management; **InfC** = Infection Control; **Efcy** = Efficacy; **Appr** = Appropriateness; **Avail** = Availability; **Timl** = Timeliness; **Efct** = Effectiveness; **Cont** = Continuity; **Safe** = Safety; **Efcn** = Efficiency; **RspC** = Respect and Caring; **JCAHO** = JCAHO Required; **ExtC** = External Comparison; **StReq** = State Required; **Status** = Not Met (N) • Met (M) • Exceeded (E).

MEASURES	IDS	SCE	ClinO	PS-S	PatSat	CostEff	PatOut	OutS	EmD	HHC	OH	CritC	PRgt	PAss	CarePt	PFEd	ContC	Lead	EnvC	HR	InfoM	InfC	Efcy	Appr	Avail	Timl	Efct	Cont	Safe	Efcn	RspC	JCAHO	ExtC	StReq	Status
Readmission Rate			X		X	X	X				X	X			X	X	X							X											M
Unsched. Readmit Rate			X		X	X	X	X			X	X			X	X	X										X								E
Amb. Surg. Unsched. Admit			X		X	X	X								X	X	X											X							E
Surgical Wound Infection			X		X	X	X	X	X		X	X			X	X	X					X				X			X						M
Falls Resulting in Injury			X		X	X	X		X		X	X			X	X	X												X						M
AMA Without Being Seen			X		X	X	X								X	X	X							X		X									M
Nosocomial Infection Rate			X		X	X	X	X	X		X	X			X	X	X					X							X						M
IV Catheter Infection			X		X	X	X	X				X			X	X	X					X							X						M
Cancelled Amb. Surgs.			X		X	X	X	X	X		X				X	X	X							X											M
Mortality/Morbidity			X		X	X	X	X			X	X			X	X	X										X								M
Merge/Joint Venture	X																	X										X							M
Expand Ambulatory Svcs.	X										X							X												X					E
Home Health Care Growth	X									X								X										X							M
Physicians On-line	X				X																X														N
Cost per Discharge		X				X		X										X								X	X								M
Safety Statistics		X				X													X							X	X		X	X					M
Cost per Amb. Surgery		X				X		X		X								X												X	X				M
Patient Satisfaction					X																										X				

MEASURES	IDS	SCE	ClinO	PS-S	PatSat	CostEff	PatOut	OutS	EmD	HHC	OH	CritC	PRgt	PAss	CarePt	PFEd	ContC	Lead	EnvC	HR	InfoM	InfC	Efcy	Appr	Avail	Timl	Efct	Cont	Safe	Efcn	RspC	JCAHO	ExtC	StReq	Status
Unscheduled Returns/OR			X		X	X	X	X			X			X	X	X											X								M
Quit Smoke Program			X		X	X	X				X			X	X	X		X									X	X							N
Cardiac Rehab			X								X			X	X	X	X							X	X			X							N

Exhibit 5.3 Progress Communication and Planning

Recommended Reading

Administrative partners plan delivers big savings. 1995. *Patient-Focused Care.* October: 112–115.

Aliotta, S. 1995. Case management programs: Investment in the future. *HMO Practice.* December: 174–178.

Coffey, R. et al. 1993. Asking effective questions: An important leadership role to support quality improvement. *The Joint Commission Journal on Quality Improvement.* October: 454–464.

Elliott, L. 1996. Integrating quality assurance and continuous quality improvement. *Surgical Services Management.* August: 45–46.

Fama, T., and P. Fox. 1995. Beyond the benefit package. *HMO Practice.* December: 179–181.

Geehr, E. 1992. The search for what works. *Healthcare Forum Journal.* July/August: 28–33.

Hospital finds success with CM (case management) approach on second try—emphasis now on outcomes. 1994. *Hospital Case Management.* February: 21–26.

Ollier, C. 1996. At 940-bed Hartford Hospital, collaboration is key to quality and culture gains, plus $50 million in savings. *Strategies for Healthcare Excellence.* January: 1–8.

Oversight team keeps CQI tied to strategic mission. 1995. *QI/TQM. January: 9–12.*

Rind, D. 1994. Effect of computer-based alerts on the treatment and outcomes of hospitalized patients. *Archives of Internal Medicine.* July 11: 1,511–1,517.

Schall, M. 1996. Innovative approaches to demand management. *Quality Connection.* Winter: 10–11.

Appendix A
Process Management Tools

For

- **Facilitators**
- **Team leaders**
- **Managers**
  - *Performance & process improvement*
  - *Management responsibilities*
  - *Team problem solving*

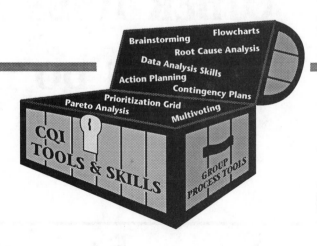

GROUP PROCESS TOOLS ARE JUST LIKE ANY OTHER TOOL

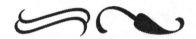

SOMETIMES, IT TAKES EVERY TOOL IN THE BOX TO FIX A PROBLEM, OTHER TIMES A HAMMER CAN DO IT ALL

Introduction

Think of your worst recurring problem. The problem that eats up your day, won't go away, and when it does, you know it's just a matter of time until it comes back again. Lost dentures, call-ins, late medical records, difficult to place patients, long waiting times, and lost requisitions are just a few of the hundreds of time-chomping problems that could be prevented… if only you had time. Now, think about what life would be like if that problem was solved. Think about the joy of coming to work and focusing solely on doing the right thing the right way. Think about the time that you could call your own again. If you're a working manager in a health-care organization, you probably work more than a 40-hour week, so that time could be coming back to you in a very personal way. That is what the scientific method, the **Performance Improvement Action Path**, can do for you.

With the help of group process tools, teams can solve problems, prevent problems, and achieve breakthroughs that continue to amaze even the most cynical among us. It's not a fad. If it were, it would be gone by now. Giving the power to subject matter experts—so they can study the process and improve performance results—has a predictable track record for success.

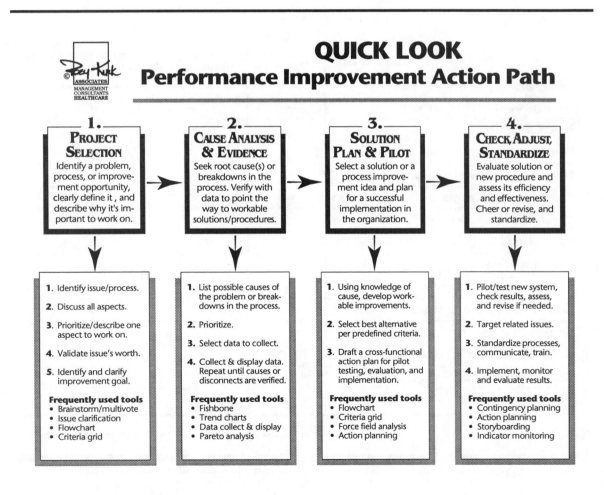

QUICK LOOK
Performance Improvement Action Path

1. PROJECT SELECTION	**2. CAUSE ANALYSIS & EVIDENCE**	**3. SOLUTION PLAN & PILOT**	**4. CHECK, ADJUST, STANDARDIZE**
Identify a problem, process, or improvement opportunity, clearly define it , and describe why it's important to work on.	Seek root cause(s) or breakdowns in the process. Verify with data to point the way to workable solutions/procedures.	Select a solution or a process improvement idea and plan for a successful implementation in the organization.	Evaluate solution or new procedure and assess its efficiency and effectiveness. Cheer or revise, and standardize.

1. Identify issue/process.	1. List possible causes of the problem or breakdowns in the process.	1. Using knowledge of cause, develop workable improvements.	1. Pilot/test new system, check results, assess, and revise if needed.
2. Discuss all aspects.	2. Prioritize.	2. Select best alternative per predefined criteria.	2. Target related issues.
3. Prioritize/describe one aspect to work on.	3. Select data to collect.	3. Draft a cross-functional action plan for pilot testing, evaluation, and implementation.	3. Standardize processes, communicate, train.
4. Validate issue's worth.	4. Collect & display data. Repeat until causes or disconnects are verified.		4. Implement, monitor and evaluate results.
5. Identify and clarify improvement goal.			
Frequently used tools • Brainstorm/multivote • Issue clarification • Flowchart • Criteria grid	**Frequently used tools** • Fishbone • Trend charts • Data collect & display • Pareto analysis	**Frequently used tools** • Flowchart • Criteria grid • Force field analysis • Action planning	**Frequently used tools** • Contingency planning • Action planning • Storyboarding • Indicator monitoring

Do you always have to use the entire scientific method? No. If you can solve a problem by just using a flowchart, brainstorming, or a success plan, by all means do so. However, if that problem keeps coming back at you, it's an indication that you've assumed the wrong root cause and applied the wrong solution. More investigation is needed.

Why do they call the group of process techniques tools? Because of their similarity to your toolbox at home. When something breaks in your home, you go to the toolbox to get help to fix the problem. Sometimes one tool will fix it and other times you have to use them all and rebuild from scratch. Some of your tools are very versatile (the hammer can do a lot), such as brainstorming, flowcharting, and multivoting. Others are very specific to a task. Issue Clarification, for one, is only used in one phase of the scientific process. Process tools and hardware tools are used for the same purpose. The only difference is the addition of a team of subject matter experts.

WHEN RESULTS MOVE OUTSIDE THE ACCEPTABLE RANGE OR YOU JUST DECIDE IT'S TIME TO CONTINUE IMPROVING...

Performance Improvement Action Path

PROCESS STEP / TOOLS	1. PROJECT SELECTION	2. CAUSE ANALYSIS	3. SOLUTION PLAN & PILOT	4. CHECK, ADJUST, STANDARDIZE
BRAINSTORMING & MULTIVOTING	**X**	X	X	X
ISSUE CLARIFICATION	**X**			
FLOWCHART (Time Sequenced, Detailed, Top-down, Matrix)	**X**	X	**X**	X
ISHAKAWA'S FISHBONE DIAGRAM	X	**X**		
TREND (OR RUN) CHARTS	X	**X**		**X**
DATA COLLECTION TOOLS (Surveys, Sampling, Checksheets)	X	**X**		**X**
DATA DISPLAY TOOLS (Trend, Pie, Bar Charts, Checksheets)	X	**X**		
PARETO ANALYSIS	X	**X**		
CRITERIA GRID AND COST-BENEFIT ANALYSIS	**X**		**X**	
LEWIN'S FORCE FIELD ANALYSIS			**X**	X
SUCCESS PLANNING			**X**	**X**
ACTION PLANNING & RECORDING	X	X	**X**	**X**
STORYBOARDING			X	**X**
INDICATOR MONITORING	X		**X**	**X**

X - Recommended tool for this step   X - Frequently useful for this step

Why are the tools necessary? Team members and sometimes the leaders are very close, and sometimes emotional, about the issue. It is not unusual for the team leader to have to manage conflict, anger, and a lot of judging and blaming. There's no way around it if subject matter experts need to be involved. And they must because it is they who have the answers. Using a process management tool and a flipchart keeps all the members of the team visually and intellectually focused on the issue, instead of on each other. Second, the tools help the team leader keep the group focused on the topic at hand. Getting off on tangents is a major cause of breakdown in teams, and the tools are the first and best way to manage the flow. Third, working on a flipchart leaves a written record of the team's decisions, which can be used for minutes, storyboards, and a reminder to the members that a particular issue has already been addressed and consensus has been reached. They are management tools and can (and should) be used any time a group is responsible for a consensus-based decision.

How do I know which tool to use when? Initially, use the toolbox guide on the previous page. As the team pursues each phase of the scientific method, look down the corresponding column to see which tools are recommended (bold X) and which ones might also work. Another alternative is to look at the guide on the bottom of the tool. If you love flowcharting, for example, and you've just defined the project, you'll be happy to know that you can also use flowcharting to seek out and verify the root cause of the problem. Finally, as you become more familiar with the tools, you'll develop a sense of what works well in certain situations. You'll also have personal preferences, so trust your intuition and experience.

What if the tool I select doesn't work? Be honest. Tell the team the tool isn't working, or that you've hit a dead end. If the team agrees, suggest another tool. Many times, however, when team members have something of value to contribute, it manages to get out on the table, regardless of the tool used.

Information about this guide. On each of the following tool pages, there is some basic information about the tool, what it's used for, and when to use the tool. Next, there are step-by-step instructions for using the tool, an example or two, and some additional hints and information about the tool. Following the toolbox section are blank copies of the tools. However, a word of caution is offered. The blank tools are recommended for documentation and storyboard purposes, not for group work. Working on a flipchart is the best way to facilitate group input for several reasons: (1) Everyone can see what is being discussed, (2) everyone sees the same thing, (3) the physical focus is on the issue, not on team members and personalities, and (4) a written record is generated that gives the team an immediate reference and also helps with documenting the team actions and decisions for the minutes.

Action Plan

What   A sequenced list (by priority or time) of results to be achieved, supported by a list of specific **activities, processes, resources,** and accountabilities that **ensure** the desired **results.**

Use for
- **Planning** significant or complex activities, particularly one that will generate change
- **Implementing** a problem solution or improvement idea
- Meeting **minutes**

When
- There's a lot to do and a schedule with **accountability** is needed.
- The group has a goal but lacks a plan for achieving it.
- **Support** from other people or departments is needed.

Directions for use
Action Plan

Many great solutions and improvement ideas are lost at the point of implementation. Planning for implementation **with key players and involved departments can prevent the loss. For each desired result ask:**

1. What are the **expected results?**

2. **How** will results be accomplished?

3. What **resources** (labor, equipment, supplies, money) will be needed?

4. How will **results** be **measured?**

5. What is the target **completion date?**

6. Who will be **responsible** for results?

Action Planning Form

Objective What are the expected results?	Action How will results be accomplished? Specifically, what steps will be taken?	Resources needed & their cost (Labor, supplies, equipment)	Indicator How will results be measured?	• Completion Date (When) • Responsible Person (Who)
• **Empowered employees:** 　- **Build teams** 　- **Develop skills** 　- **Delegate** 　- **Let go**	• Involve staff and reach mutual agreement on goals • Tell participants 　- Why job is important 　- Why it needs to be done 　- Why they were chosen • Delegate in terms of result... but let them decide how • Define authority and constraints before they start • Plan controls, schedule specific, timely feedback	• 2 hours every other week for meetings	**Standard:** Employees actively participate in CQI process. **Indicator:** 4 departmental problems solved annually (2 chosen by employees, 2 chosen by dept. manager)	• Department manager • 80% of department employees

PS   CA   SP   CAS

Brainstorming

What　First used by Walt Disney, made famous by advertising wizard Alex Osborn, the once free-for-all calling out of ideas is now used in a more methodical, **structured** format to **generate a list of ideas** on almost any topic or issue.

Use for　Creating a list of ideas/issues:
- **Problems,** processes to fix, or improvement **opportunities**
- **Data** to collect and analyze
- **Solutions** and improvements
- Significant **indicators** to monitor

When
- **Multiple ideas** are needed.
- Group is **stuck**/low energy.
- Sufficient time is available.

Directions for use
Brainstorming

1. **Select a topic to brainstorm (B/S).**

   - *Clarify topic and available time (should relate to issue importance).*
   - *Keep it focused for best results.*
   - *Allow the group some "think" time.*

2. **Offer ideas in turn, recording <u>all</u> on a flipchart everyone can see.**

   - *Pass if you don't have an idea.*
   - *Build on brainstormed ideas.*
   - *No evaluation of ideas allowed. Even positive comments interrupt the flow of ideas and slow the process.*

3. **B/S until ideas are exhausted. Don't be discouraged by several rounds of passing. One new idea often sparks fresh rounds of other ideas.**

4. **Always multivote a brainstormed list.**

Example
Brainstorming

Brainstorm list: Desired characteristics for facilitators & team leaders

1. Performance rated high – Walk-the-talk
2. Sense of humor
3. Bright future in organization
4. People skills: Likes, and is liked by others
5. Optimistic outlook
6. Willing to share recognition, control
7. Able to remain neutral or step aside
8. Manage conflict, confrontation, defensiveness
9. High energy and stamina
10. Self-confident but not arrogant
11. Credible and respected
12. Organizational knowledge, experience
13. Enthusiastic about task
14. Flexible and open-minded
15. Likes (or at least tolerates) change
16. Creative
17. Sends clear, concise messages
18. Risks and learns from mistakes/successes
19. Asks questions and listens to answers
20. _____

Alternatives and tips

1. *Give the group adequate time to think before you begin the brainstorm session. This can vary from as little as a few minutes to several days.*

2. *Wallstorming really works!*

   - *Tape 8–10 flipchart sheets up around a room that has room for walking (double layer for wall protection).*
   - *Offer one broad topic or subtopic on the individual sheets.*
   - *Give everyone a marker and let them walk off lunch or pace while they ponder the issue(s) at hand.*

3. *Brainstorm on Post-it™ notes.*

   - *Saves writing time for team leader.*
   - *Group by topic for an affinity diagram, put in chronological order for a flowchart, or attach to a fishbone diagram.*

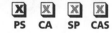
PS　CA　SP　CAS

Checksheets

What A dual method for both **collecting** data and **displaying data** in a meaningful and easy-to-understand format.

Use for
- Analyzing a problem's **root causes**
- **Gathering data**
- Providing an easy-to-understand record of data gathered
- Giving a visual **illustration** of what is happening

When
- **Several people** are collecting data that will later be combined.
- Perceptions need to be backed up by **hard data**.
- You need to **sell** an **audience** who is unfamiliar with issues & data.

Directions for use
Checksheets

1. **Decide data to be observed or collected and a realistic time period for analysis.**

2. **Design a form on which to record data, making sure it's clear and easy to use so data collection will be standardized.**

3. **Pilot form with an unfamiliar but feedback-friendly group. Revise if needed.**

4. **Decide how data will be collected.**

5. **Combine information on a master tally and draw the graphic.**

   - *Simple tabulation*
   - *Visual checksheet*
   - *Matrix checksheet*
   - *Symbol checksheet*

Examples

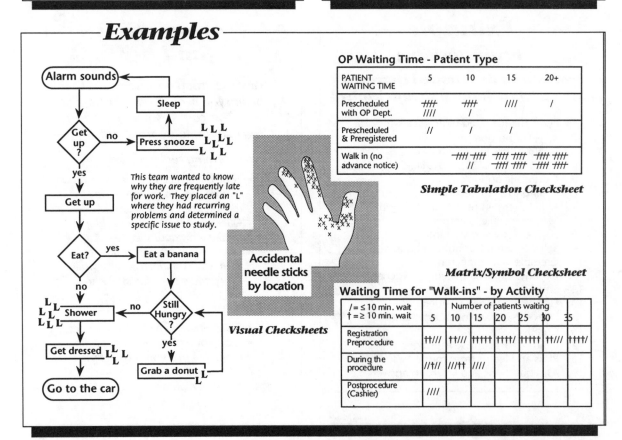

This team wanted to know why they are frequently late for work. They placed an "L" where they had recurring problems and determined a specific issue to study.

Visual Checksheets

Accidental needle sticks by location

OP Waiting Time - Patient Type

PATIENT WAITING TIME	5	10	15	20+
Prescheduled with OP Dept.	＃＃＃ ////	＃＃＃ /	////	/
Prescheduled & Preregistered	//	/	/	
Walk in (no advance notice)		＃＃＃ ＃＃＃ //	＃＃＃ ＃＃＃ ＃＃＃ ＃＃＃	＃＃＃ ＃＃＃ ＃＃＃ ＃＃＃

Simple Tabulation Checksheet

Matrix/Symbol Checksheet

Waiting Time for "Walk-ins" - by Activity

/ = ≤ 10 min. wait † = ≥ 10 min. wait	Number of patients waiting						
	5	10	15	20	25	30	35
Registration Preprocedure	††///	††///	†††††/	†††††/	†††††	††///	†††††/
During the procedure	//†//	///††	////				
Postprocedure (Cashier)	////						

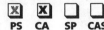

PS CA SP CAS

Cost-Benefit Analysis

What A method of comparing/analyzing two or more alternatives to determine which one produces the **best return on investment**. Both costs and potential benefits are considered.

Use to
- **Evaluate** two or more **solutions**.
- Show the **cost-effectiveness** of a decision.
- Put a **dollar value** on **benefits**.
- Evaluate an option financially.

When
- **Indecision** exists between two solutions or options.
- A selected solution seems too expensive, but clearly gives the **best return on investment**.
- The **cost-effectiveness** of an option needs to be demonstrated.

Directions for use
Cost-Benefit Analysis

1. Decide **analysis period** (year, month, etc.).

2. For each option, brainstorm all related **costs**. Then research* and reach consensus on the dollar value of each cost listed and **total** the "tangible costs" for each option.

3. For each option, brainstorm all related **benefits**. Research and reach consensus on the dollar value of each. Then **total** the "tangible benefits costs" for each option.

$$\frac{\text{Benefits}}{\text{Costs}} = \text{Cost-Benefit Ratio}$$

4. To determine **cost-benefit ratio**, apply formula to each option. The larger the number, the better the return on investment (benefit dollars returned per dollar spent to change).

---

* Consult purchasing, finance, and other experts for input on costs. Have detail available to back up dollar assessment if using cost-benefit to gain support from senior management for a proposed solution.

Option #1 or

Buy a new computer		1 year	
PROPOSED SOLUTION OR OPTION		ANALYSIS PERIOD	

TANGIBLE COSTS	DOLLAR VALUE	TANGIBLE BENEFITS	DOLLAR VALUE
• Hardware	$10,000	• Delete .5 clerk	$6,000
• Software/supplies	1,200	• Dollars saved by in-house printing capability	$9,000
• Training	$4,000		
• Planning	$1,500	• Increase new products (5) developed	$25,000
• Start-up	$3,000		
	$19,700		$40,000

INTANGIBLE COSTS	INTANGIBLE BENEFITS
• Down time	• Professional-looking work
• Resistance to the new technology by staff members	• Convenience
	• Reduction of proposal turnaround and increase in market share

$$\frac{\text{Benefits}}{\text{Costs}} = \text{Cost Benefit Ratio} \qquad \frac{40,000}{19,700} = 2.03$$

Option #2

Hire full-time secretary		1 year	
PROPOSED SOLUTION OR OPTION		ANALYSIS PERIOD	

TANGIBLE COSTS	DOLLAR VALUE	TANGIBLE BENEFITS	DOLLAR VALUE
• Salary	$15,000	• Delete .5 clerk	$6,000
• Benefits	$4,500	• Answer phone	$3,000
• Orient/train	$1,200	• Increase new products (2) developed	$10,000
• Desk/supplies	$1,900		
• Start-up	$3,000		$19,000
	$25,600		

INTANGIBLE COSTS	INTANGIBLE BENEFITS
• High rate of turnover	• Easy to access
• Underutilization	• Convenience
• Domino-effect. Other departments will want one.	• Reliability in work completion

$$\frac{\text{Benefits}}{\text{Costs}} = \text{Cost Benefit Ratio} \qquad \frac{19,000}{25,600} = .74$$

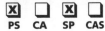

☒	☐	☒	☐
PS	CA	SP	CAS

Criteria Grid

What A tool that uses **predetermined criteria** to **prioritize** and narrow down a selection of ideas to just one preference.

Use for Selecting just one from a list of options. These options might be:

- A **problem** to study and fix
- An **improvement** opportunity
- A **process** to improve
- A **solution** to apply

When
- A group is **unable to reach consensus** with discussion alone.
- There is **bias** or **lack of information**-based decision making in the group.

A.K.A. Selection Grid or Prioritization Matrix

Directions for use
Criteria Grid

1. Identify 3 to 4 issues (can be taken from multivoting results) for the grid.

2. Select or brainstorm relevant criteria (3–6 max.) and scoring mechanism (yes/no, high/medium/low, 1–5 scale).

3. Have group evaluate each option in light of criteria. Data can be collected by hands up voting or ballots.

4. When complete, evaluate findings and reach consensus on best option.

- Does one option meet all criteria?
- Is more than one option acceptable?
- Should any options be eliminated?
- If an option meets most of the criteria, but not all, should it still be considered?
- Overall, which option seems best?

Criteria Grid Example
Emergency Dept. Delays

EVALUATION CRITERIA →

↓ **ISSUE TO PRIORITIZE**

Potential Projects

	Enough time? Yes (Y) or No (N)	Mgt. support? Yes (Y) or No (N)	Right members? Yes (Y) or No (N)	Team enthusiasm High (H) Med (M) Low (L)	Return on invest? High (H) Med (M) Low (L)
ED patient waiting time	Y = 2 N = 8	Y = 5 N = 5	Y = 7 N = 3	H = 10 M = 0 L = 0	H = 2 M = 6 L = 2
Unit scheduling problems	Y = 9 N = 1	Y = 10 N = 0	Y = 10 N = 0	H = 6 M = 4 L = 0	H = 0 M = 6 L = 4
Standing physician orders	Y = 2 N = 8	Y = 3 N = 7	Y = 0 N = 10	H = 10 M = 0 L = 0	H = 8 M = 1 L = 1

This team chose "Scheduling Problems" to work on, even though it wasn't an interest priority because they had the time, management support, and the right team members. It was the best option for now, but they planned to start building physician awareness and support so they could work on the "orders" issue next.

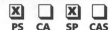

PS CA SP CAS

Criteria Grid Example
Employee Satisfaction

EVALUATION CRITERIA →

↓ **ISSUE TO PRIORITIZE**

Potential solutions	Can we control? Yes (Y) or No (N)	Team/mgt. support? Yes (Y) or No (N)	Cost-to-benefit ratio Benefit ÷ Costs	Employee requested High (H) Med (M) Low (L)	System support? High (H) Med (M) Low (L)		
Offer flexible scheduling options to all depts.	Y = 2 N = 8	Y = 3 N = 7	.9	H = 10 M = 0 L = 0	H = 2 M = 6 L = 2		
Revamp of performance evaluation system	Y = 1 N = 9	Y = 10 N = 0	1.5	H = 6 M = 4 L = 0	H = 0 M = 6 L = 4		
Employees are involved in departmental decisions	Y = 8 N = 2	Y = 5 N = 5	2.1	H = 10 M = 0 L = 0	H = 8 M = 1 L = 1		

Problem Criteria

Groups often get stuck trying to select criteria. Suggestions follow, but remember every situation is different and may need unique criteria. And some criteria can be used for both problems and solutions. Usually, teams brainstorm a list and then narrow it down to 3 or 4 by multivoting.

Time – Is there enough to do justice to this issue?

Timeliness/urgency – Is it the right time? Do we have to resolve other issues before this one?

Doable – Is it possible to achieve what we'd like?

Management support – Is there support to work on this issue? Don't assume, ask them.

Interest – Is there team support and enthusiasm and a belief that it is worthwhile?

Influence/control – Are we the right people?

Important – Will it matter if we get great results? Is the impact on clinical, customer service, or financial outcomes?

Resources – Do we have enough people, supplies, time, money, and equipment to pursue this issue? Is this a resource priority?

Solution Criteria

Return on investment/Cost-to-benefit ratio – Is there a payoff (financial or benefit) potential?

Timeliness/urgency – Is it the right time? Can we complete within a set time frame?

Doable – Can this be implemented successfully?

Team/management support – Is there support for the implementation of this solution?

Employee preferred – Will our key customers be pleased and satisfied with this solution?

Influence/control – Do we have it? Are we the right people to implement this solution?

Visible – To what extent will this solution and its results be seen and scrutinized by others?

Resources – Do we have enough resources to pursue this issue? Is this a resource priority?

☒ PS ☐ CA ☒ SP ☐ CAS

Data Collection

What A way to back up and **document** assumptions and perceptions about **performance results** with actual information or data.

Use for
- Comparing actual **outcome** and **process** results to preset targets
- Targeting potential improvement **opportunities**
- Determining if a **team** is **needed**
- **Illustrating** what is happening

When
- **Routine** quality assessment
- As needed, to look at **unstable** outcomes or processes
- **Recurring** or common cause problems, cross-functional processes

Questions to ask
for successful data collection

- ❑ What information do you need and what data do you need to collect?
- ❑ Have the data already been collected? Are they available? Accessible?
- ❑ Are the data timely enough? Relevant?
- ❑ Is the sample size* adequate?
- ❑ Is the form standardized? Has it been tested for efficiency and reliability?

---

*A guideline from Joint Commission–
"If the average number of cases per quarter is more than 600, at least 5% of cases are reviewed; and If the average number of cases per quarter is fewer than 600, at least 30 cases are reviewed."[1]

Data tools

Can be used to:	Collect	Display	Analyze
■ Surveys (written, phone, interview)	x		x
■ Fishbone diagram	x		
■ Sampling	x		
■ Observation	x		
■ Task or checklists	x		
■ Checksheets	x	x	x
■ Cost-benefit analysis	x	x	x
■ Run (a.k.a. trend)		x	x
■ Pie and bar charts		x	x
■ Control charts		x	x
■ Histograms	x	x	x
■ Scatter diagrams		x	x
■ Pareto diagrams		x	x
■ Flowcharts	x	x	x

Data reminders and thoughts

- ❑ First, decide what data or information you need. That will help you select the best way to collect and display.
- ❑ Make sure data collection forms are standardized and piloted.
- ❑ Let others involved know why you are collecting the data and what will be done with the information.
- ❑ Offer to share collected information when the project is complete.
- ❑ If you can't measure it, you can't manage it. – Anonymous
- ❑ Torture the data long enough and they will confess to anything. – Anonymous

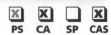

PS CA SP CAS

Data Presentation

A *picture* really is worth a thousand words, so when you have to present, make sure you present pictures... not numbers!

Pie charts
Display 100% of the data as well as individual percentages and their relationship to the total

Column and bar charts
Allow comparisons among data and sometimes show a particular pattern (Pareto and histograms)

Run (or trend) charts
Illustrate performance results **over time** or how a process performs **over time**

Pie Charts

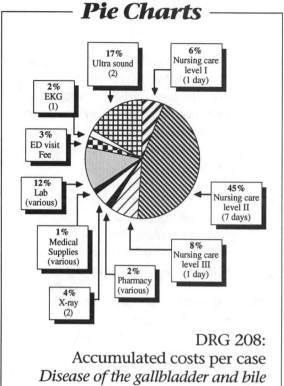

DRG 208:
Accumulated costs per case
Disease of the gallbladder and bile

Column & Bar Charts

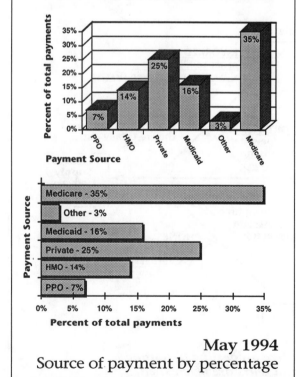

May 1994
Source of payment by percentage

Run/Trend Charts

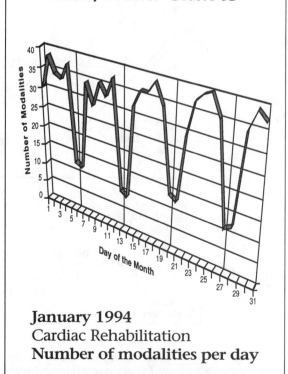

January 1994
Cardiac Rehabilitation
Number of modalities per day

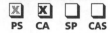

PS   CA   SP   CAS

Fishbone

What A brainstormed diagram of **possible "root" causes** of a **recurring problem**. The goal is to get increasingly more specific so the group can reach **consensus** on a potential "cause," then **collect data** to back up their perception.

Use for
• Extracting **experiential knowledge** from a group
• Sparking creativity
• Building on others' ideas
• Reaching group consensus

When
• **Identify** and **clarify** problem.
• Target possible root causes.
• Identify **key data** to collect.

***

Originator: **Kaoru Ishikawa**

Directions for use
Fishbone Diagram

1. On a flipchart, draw an arrow diagram as below.

2. Label main bones. Use **procedures, people, materials, measurements,** and **equipment** (or any key words that might inspire creative thinking).

3. Brainstorm <u>possible</u> root causes (see reference for steps).

   • Pursue subcauses by asking "Why."

   • Build on others' ideas.

4. Multivote to reach consensus, and prioritize possible root causes (see multivote tool page for steps).

5. Identify the data that will verify the team's assumptions of root cause and then proceed to data collection.

Example

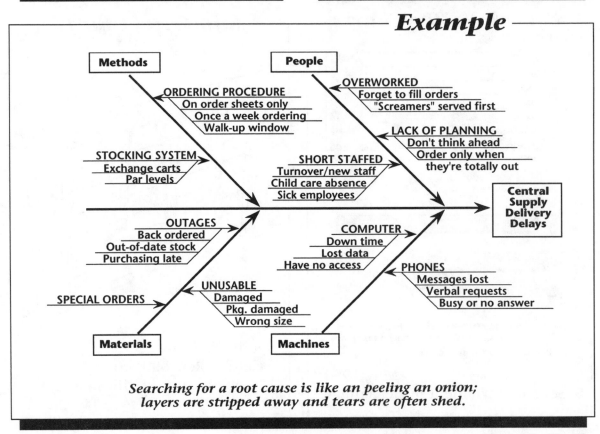

Searching for a root cause is like an peeling an onion; layers are stripped away and tears are often shed.

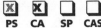

PS   CA   SP   CAS

Flowchart

What   An *illustration* of a work process including all activities & decisions.

Use for
- *Identifying all action steps and decisions within a process*
- *Highlighting problem areas in in the process (disconnects, bottlenecks, mysteries)*
- *Creating agreement on how the process can be improved and should work – leading to a standard operating procedure*

When
- *A process isn't working, "blaming" is rampant, and a root cause(s) needs to be discovered.*
- *Streamlining processes.*
- *Solution implementation planning.*
- *Clinical or ideal service path design.*

Directions for use
Flowchart

1. **Convene a group of people who participate in and own the process.**

2. **Reach consensus on where the process begins and ends.**

3. **Brainstorm activities and decisions in the process (in any order).**

4. **Create chart: Put activities and decisions in their current order (this may be painful). Use arrows to show direction of flow.**

   - *Break down complex activities as needed (may occur outside team).*

   - *Identify the pain (disconnects, bottlenecks, mysteries).*

   - *Reach consensus on improving and streamlining the process.*

Example

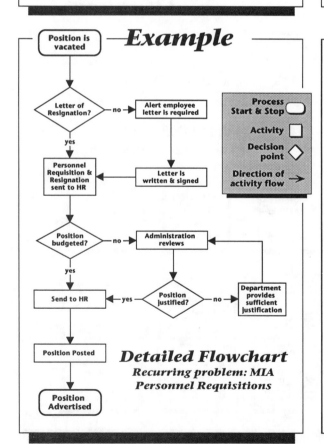

Detailed Flowchart
Recurring problem: MIA Personnel Requisitions

Extra Hints

- *Process analysis can get <u>very</u> complex quickly, so look at the big picture first. Deeper looks can occur at future meetings or outside the team.*

- *Brainstorm each activity or decision on its own Post-it™ note. (Different colors or shapes can be used to distinguish decisions from activities or department responsibility.) Groups rarely have immediate consensus on order. Movable notes provide flexibility in both drafting the chart and improving the process later on.*

- *Use multivoting to identify where the process is breaking down or disconnecting.*

- *Look for opportunities to streamline the process. Preventing turnover, in the example, could have eliminated this flowchart all together.*

PS   CA   SP   CAS

Flowchart (continued)

Flowchart & Checksheet

Recurring problem: Delays causing increased waits in outpatient services

Multivote prioritizes the bottlenecks & breakdowns

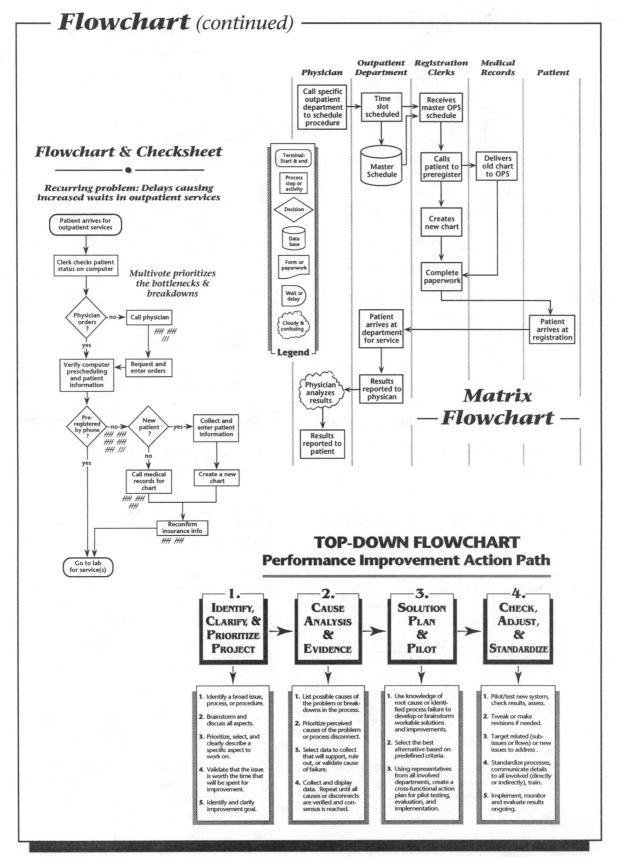

Matrix — Flowchart —

TOP-DOWN FLOWCHART
Performance Improvement Action Path

1. IDENTIFY, CLARIFY, & PRIORITIZE PROJECT	2. CAUSE ANALYSIS & EVIDENCE	3. SOLUTION PLAN & PILOT	4. CHECK, ADJUST, & STANDARDIZE
1. Identify a broad issue, process, or procedure.	1. List possible causes of the problem or break-downs in the process.	1. Use knowledge of root cause or identi-fied process failure to develop or brainstorm workable solutions and improvements.	1. Pilot/test new system, check results, assess.
2. Brainstorm and discuss all aspects.	2. Prioritize perceived causes of the problem or process disconnect.	2. Select the best alternative based on predefined criteria.	2. Tweak or make revisions if needed.
3. Prioritize, select, and clearly describe a specific aspect to work on.	3. Select data to collect that will support, rule out, or validate cause of failure.	3. Using representatives from all involved departments, create a cross-functional action plan for pilot testing, evaluation, and implementation.	3. Target related (sub-issues or flows) or new issues to address.
4. Validate that the issue is worth the time that will be spent for improvement.	4. Collect and display data. Repeat until all causes or disconnects are verified and con-sensus is reached.		4. Standardize processes, communicate details to all involved (directly or indirectly), train.
5. Identify and clarify improvement goal.			5. Implement, monitor and evaluate results ongoing.

PS CA SP CAS

Force Field Analysis
Source: Kurt Lewin

What An interactive process for **planning** and identifying, ahead of time, **existing forces that impact** (1) goal achievement, (2) solution implementation, and (3) risk minimization.

Use for
- **Evaluating** whether a **solution** or goal is realistic and achievable
- Proactively identifying **obstacles to** successful implementation
- Facilitating interactive planning, **communication, participation**
- Involving key process participants
- **Reducing resistance** to change

When
- Resistance is present (rampant).
- All key players have not been directly involved with the team.
- The **implementation** is complex.

Directions for use
Force Field

1. **Draw the Force Field "T" on a flipchart: Current situation in the center and proposed solution or goal to the right.**

2. **Brainstorm (see tool page for steps).**

   - Resisting forces or <u>existing</u> <u>obstacles</u> to successful implementation.

   - <u>Existing</u> <u>forces</u> or circumstances that will help achieve the desired state. Note: negative circumstances can and often are driving forces.

3. **Multivote (see tool page for steps).**

   - Prioritize both sides of chart.

   - Action plan to remove obstacles before you start to implement.

   - Action plan to use driving forces to your advantage in implementing.

Example

Force Field Analysis	Current State	Goal/Solution
	Zero time to myself	1 hour each day

Driving Forces Existing circumstances helping us achieve our desired goal/solution	Resisting Forces Existing forces (obstacles) keeping us from achieving our desired goal/solution
No fun/Depressed	So much work ✝✝✝ //
Not enjoying work	(Shared secretary) ✝✝✝ ✝✝✝
Low productivity	Budget cutbacks ✝✝✝ //
Miss tennis pals	Never feel done
5-pound gain	Family pressures
No exercise time	Unmotivated
Journal piles	Love my job ✝✝✝

Remove Obstacles
Success Plan

I have to share a secretary who is never available when needed.

WRITE GOAL RESULT, PROBLEM, <u>OR</u> ISSUE ABOVE

1. How can I ensure inadequate clerical support? TO FAIL	2. How can I complete all clerical responsibilities? TO SUCCEED
• Avoid computers --->>	• Get a computer
• Be a martyr --------->>	• No way. No payoff!
• Get a bigger briefcase & take more work home	• Plan to limit hours and homework
• Don't schedule or plan for secretarial needs	• Preschedule & plan for secretarial needs
• Do everything myself, never delegate	• Plan & train to delegate when possible
• Don't document or analyze workload	• Document & analyze clerical workload
• Learn to type faster	• Hand notes & voicemail

PS CA SP CAS

Histogram

What   Repeated events will always produce results that vary over time. A histogram displays the **pattern of that variation**, as well as the frequency and extent of the variation.

Use for   • Measuring **how frequently** a situation (desired outcome, problem, error, breakdown, etc.) occurs.

   • Displaying the **distribution** of data with a bar chart.

   • Analyzing and interpreting data and how they are distributed.

When   • A lot of data need to be displayed in a meaningful and useful way.

   • To determine if performance is conforming to a normal distribution.

Directions for use

1. Collect the data. A minimum of 30 is recommended.

2. Count the number of data points in the data set (e.g. N=32).

3. Sort and tally the data.

4. Determine the range (R) by subtracting the lowest value from the highest.

5. For horizontal axis points, divide the range into classes (5–7 classes for 50 or less points, 6–10 for 50–100 points).

6. Determine the cell width (H) by dividing the range (R) by the classes (K).

7. Tally all occurrences in each cell, construct the histogram, and tally.

8. Remember, the goal is to find a situation that stands out (an abnormal distribution or a Pareto distribution).

Example

If we monitored the length of waiting time in the ER and saw the following distributions, what would they tell us?

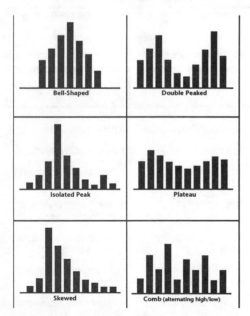

Bell-Shaped   Double Peaked
Isolated Peak   Plateau
Skewed   Comb (alternating high/low)

Interpretation*

1. **Bell-Shaped** – This is a "normal" or natural pattern of events. Reinforces the notion that 85% of occurrences will fall within a normal range of variation.

2. **Double peaked** – It is likely that two different processes are at work – different time frames, different people, different departments, etc. Experts recommend stratifying the data sample.

3. **Isolated peak** – This may be an extreme case of double peak with two distinct processes or possibly a Pareto. Again stratification may help.

4. **Plateau** – This indicates a broken or nonexistent process (everyone does their own thing). Process variation usually produces variation in results.

5. **Skewed** – The skew (long tail on right) indicates that an obstacle is at work, limiting the chances of achieving results (lower left).

6. **Comb** – Usually it has to do with how the data are broken up (perhaps the data are being sliced too many times) or that there is bias in the data.

Interpretation, without evidence, is only a theory.

PS   CA   SP   CAS

Indicator Development

What   *A way to understand our choices. We can do the **right things** or the **wrong things**. We can do them the **right way** or the **wrong way**.*

Use for • *Results and performance (process) indicator development/design*
• *Identifying **avoidable** & **necessary** costs of quality (How much of your time do you spend in the right-things-right quadrant?)*

When   • *A solution, **new process**, or improvement idea is **implemented** and needs objective measures.*
• ***Avoidable costs of quality** need to be identified and improved.*
• ***Routine** measurement is done.*

Designing Performance

*Indicators help people **plan** to do the right things the right way... all the time.*

■ *Outcome indicators - provide a desired goal or target to attain (what).*

 • ***Efficacy*** - was the outcome achieved?*

 • ***Appropriateness*** - was the care/intervention relevant to patient's needs?*

■ *Process indicators - a roadmap/recipe for attaining a desired outcome (how).*

 • *Availability**   • *Safety**

 • *Timeliness**   • *Efficiency**

 • *Effectiveness**   • *Respect & Caring**

 • *Continuity**

---
*Joint Commission's 's *Definitions of Dimensions of Performance.*[2]

Outcome & Process Indicators

Outcome or result • "Right" thing to do • Standard of care/service •	• Process or procedure • "Right" way to do it • Standard of performance
What outcome or result are we seeking (delighted customers, saved lives, improved quality of life)?	What process/procedure will we follow to ensure achieving outcomes on a routine, predictable basis?

Here are a few familiar examples

• All employees will be responsible for improving performance (documented with data) of two cross-functional processes	• Staff will actively contribute to improving their department's work process, cross-functional teamwork, personal effort, or task force
• Patient will be able to verbalize (prior to discharge) knowledge of exercise, pulse, and take home medications	• Nurse will evaluate patient's knowledge, fill in needed information, and document discharge knowledge
• Patient satisfaction assessment and rating is at least 8 on a scale of 1-10	• Employees will continually assess, respond, or explain why they cannot respond
• Medical records are available 24 hours per day, as evidenced by the number returned ≥ 1 week late	• MR clerk will verify ID, phone, and return date, review return policy, and offer a reminder call
• 4.0 hours per patient day delivered to med-surg patients, on the average	• Managers will monitor and maintain staffing at ± 2% of target throughout year

Assessing Performance

Indicators are met, not met, or exceeded.
• *Outcome indicators measure whether we are doing the right things.*
• *Process indicators monitor whether we are doing things the right way.*

Issues to resolve prior to implementation:

1. ***What** are we going to **monitor**? What data are we going to collect?*

2. *What other information do we need, and do we know where to find it?*

3. ***How** are we going to measure results? What method? To what extent?*

4. ***Who**'s responsible for monitoring?*

5. *When and **how often** will we monitor?*

6. *How will the information be **displayed**? Communicated?*

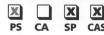

Issue Clarification

What Before a group can solve a problem or improve a process, they must clearly **define** one **specific issue** and **narrow** the focus to a workable size. Frequently, an issue is many intertwined (or cross-functional) issues.

Use for • Clarifying all aspects of the issue
 • Allowing members to **discuss** their **experiences** and viewpoints related to the issue
 • Reaching consensus and **commitment** to work on one issue
 • Confirming the issue is worth the time it will take to work on

When Each time a **new issue**, problem, or process is studied, even if it's an offshoot of a previous issue

Directions for use
Issue Clarification

1. **Today's reality.** List, then prioritize a critical or core issue to pursue.

   • What is happening with the problem or process to be improved?
   • What are the current facts?

2. **Consequence.** Discuss, list, then prioritize the ramifications of this situation and why it's worthwhile to work on.

   • So what? What's the gain for fixing?
   • Give an opportunity for war stories, venting of feelings (within a time limit)
   • Cost justify. Put a price tag on error.

3. **Improvement goal.** List, then prioritize how you'd know the problem was fixed or the process was improved.

   • Describe what success would be.
   • Target and commit to a realistic (and measurable) outcome.

Example #1
Issue Clarification

1. Today's Reality What is happening?	2. Prioritized critical or core issue: Unproductive meetings	
Broad issue A team is not achieving their anticipated results. **Sub-issues** Unproductive meetings Members are late then in and out. Interruptions (beepers/phones) Too much to do Lack of focus, tangents	**3. Consequence or Result** *Is this important?* Expensive meeting time is wasted. Decisions are not made because too many people are absent. Team's worth is questioned. Team member momentum, enthusiasm fading.	**4. Improvement Goal Desired** *A success would be...* Productive meetings and team agreement that time was well spent Issues selected impact both quality and potential cost savings. Solutions and improvement ideas have a positive cost-benefit ratio.

Note: Prioritize column 1 and use prioritized issue as a reference for completing columns 2 and 3. Include the "broad issue" in the prioritization because it may well be the best description of "what is happening."

Example #2
Issue Clarification

1. Today's Reality What is happening?	2. Prioritized critical or core issue: Most outpatients are not prescheduled or preregistered	
Broad issue Outpatient department delays **Sub-issues** Patients wait 30+ minutes for outpatient services. Most patients have not prescheduled or preregistered. OP registration clerks are overwhelmed and spend 20 minutes per patient. OP departments have no way to predict workload.	**3. Consequence or Result** *Is this important?* Patients are angry and constantly interrupt clerks, further delaying service. Departments are inadequately staffed for unknown workload. Our reputation is being damaged.	**4. Improvement Goal Desired** *A success would be...* Registration clerks will be trained to pass skills checklist. Prescheduled, preregistered patients will wait no more than 5 minutes. We will have a reputation for excellent service and draw from outside our market.

Note: Prioritize (brainstorm and multivote) all columns to avoid getting bogged down in discussion and to help reach consensus quickly.

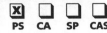

X ☐ ☐ ☐
PS CA SP CAS

Multivoting

What A method of **prioritizing** and narrowing down a list of issues. It **minimizes** the negative effects of win-lose voting, which leads to **conflict** and **polarization**.

Use for Prioritizing/narrowing any list of ideas, problems, or issues:
- Problems, processes to fix, or improvement **opportunities**
- **Data** to collect and analyze
- **Solutions** and improvements
- Significant **indicators** to monitor

When
- If there are too many issues to discuss, work on top choices.
- Group **cannot reach consensus** within a reasonable time.

Directions for use
Multivoting

1. **With group agreement, number list, clarify, and remove duplicate items.**

2. **Agree on a framework for decisions (i.e., favorite idea, most workable idea, best idea within cost constraint, etc.).**

3. **Let group briefly discuss and campaign for favored ideas. Save time to discuss top issues later.**

4. **Distribute weighting points (3–10)**

   - Leader choice: as few as 3, as many as 10, depending on time constraints and the significance of the issue.

   - Group can also take a stretch and write their own points on the flipchart.

5. **Discuss top 3–5 issues. Reach consensus on best option to pursue.**

Example
Emergency department delays

To begin reaching consensus on one issue to work on first, the team multivoted to prioritize the brainstormed list of subproblems.

1. **Patient waiting time** ~~////~~ ~~////~~ ~~////~~ ////
2. Ancillary department work delays ~~////~~ ////
3. Shortage of registration clerks ~~////~~ //
4. Admitting department ~~////~~ //
5. Patients needing outpatient services ~~////~~ //// only, coming to ED
6. **Unit scheduling problems** ~~////~~ ~~////~~ ~~////~~
7. Uncooperative families ////
8. Unable to reach/contact physicians //
9. Supply shortages ~~////~~
10. Unable to reach family for permissions ////
11. Broken/missing equipment ~~////~~ ////
12. Organizational red tape //
13. **Standing physician orders** ~~////~~ ~~////~~ ~~////~~ ////
14. Unavailable medical records ~~////~~
15. Waiting for physicians to arrive ~~////~~ //

Multivoting Quickies

Multivoting can take a lot of time, and sometimes you may just want to get a quick read of the group to test for or move the group toward consensus.

1. Number a group of ideas on a flipchart and then ask the group to say the number of their choice when you say "go." Sometimes you can hear the consensus, and the diversity. Or…

2. Review and clarify list as above. Tell the group they have 3 multivotes but can put no more than two on any one item.

   They vote by raising their hands (1 hand, 2 hands, or no hands). Going through the list this way is faster than the usual multivote procedure. Or…

3. Use the honor system and let people scribe their own multivotes.

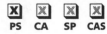

PS **CA** **SP** **CAS**

Pareto Diagram

What   Based on the Pareto Principle (80-20 Rule), it uses data collection and bar charts to spotlight the most important **source** of the problem.

Use for   • **Analyzing** a problem situation
• Backing up an assumption of **root cause** (often from a fishbone) with data
• Categorizing and **displaying data** (most frequent occurrences in descending order left to right)

When   • To **analyze routine data** collected from outcome monitoring.
• Display results that may lead to a sustainable **solution**.
• Follow up to fishbone assumptions of root cause.

Directions for use
Pareto Diagram

1. **Identify broad areas to study: when is the problem happening, where is it happening, who is it happening to, etc.**

2. **Brainstorm specific categories of data you want to collect.**

3. **Collect data and sort into the categories, displaying them in descending order (largest bar to the left) bar chart.**

   • Look for a Pareto <u>pattern</u>. Even "flat" Paretos are valuable and indicate another path should be followed.

   • You may have to do more fishbones.

4. **Sometimes a <u>perceived</u> root cause can not be validated, and it's probably the reason past solutions have failed to fix the problem.**

OPS/ED Delay Examples

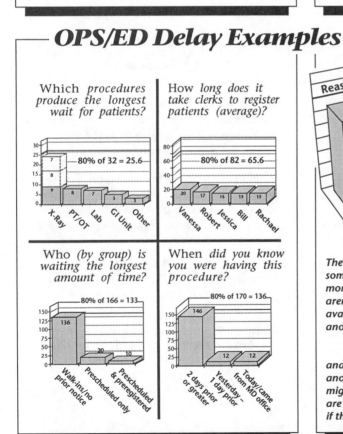

Which *procedures* produce the longest wait for patients?

How *long does it* take clerks to register patients (average)?

Who *(by group) is* waiting the longest amount of time?

When *did you know* you were having this procedure?

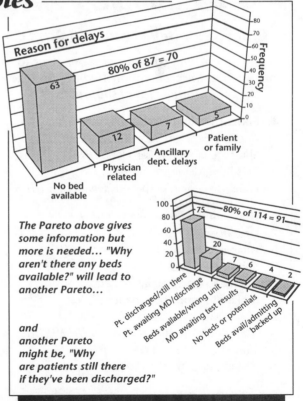

Reason for delays

The Pareto above gives some information but more is needed... "Why aren't there any beds available?" will lead to another Pareto...

and another Pareto might be, "Why are patients still there if they've been discharged?"

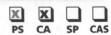

PS **CA** **SP** **CAS**

Project Checklist

***After a project or issue is selected and clarified,
compare it to this checklist to ensure getting off on the right foot.***

☑ Team **agrees** on the **project** and can clearly describe in a sentence or two (1) the issue, (2) why it needs to be addressed, and (3) the desired improvement goal.

☑ Both the team members and management believe the project and its potential payoff is **achievable** and **worth** the team's time.

☑ The project (or prioritized sub-issue) is **narrow** enough to maintain **focus.**

☑ There is **support for change** and **improvement** related to the project issues (from managers, employees, customers)

☑ Project is related (directly or indirectly) to an important **cross-functional issue.**

☑ Process is **repetitive, not in transition,** or being **studied** by another group.

☑ Current process, if one exists, is **stable** and **clearly defined** (including start/end).

☑ **Start-up projects:** Select an issue that (1) is important but uncomplicated enough to be resolved quickly, (2) showcases the value of CQI, and (3) involves those who will buy in, apply what they've learned, and champion the effort.

Opportunity Analysis

Strategic goal the project addresses _____

Specific process to be improved _____

This effort should improve _____

Key customer to be served _____

This process is important to work on now because _____

_____

_____ is the representative of this process to the PI Council.

Start date _____ Project Team is _____

Progress check dates _____ Finish date _____

Leader _____ Facilitator _____ (Attach membership list)

Constraints/instructions to the team from the Quality Council _____

_____

_____

_____

Estimated/committed team hours for the project _____

Anticipated return on investment _____ Reviewed/approved by PI Council _____

☒ ☒ ☒ ☒
PS CA SP CAS

Sampling

Random Sampling

A portion of data is selected by chance from the entire database, and each item has an equal chance of being selected. **Example:** *Pulling a name out of a fishbowl that holds 100% of employee names.*

Stratified Sampling

Data are divided into groups—an age or geographical group, a diagnosis-related group (DRG), or physician group (all surgeons)—and then each group is sampled separately using a random or systematic technique. **Example:** *Pulling randomly (or systematically) out of a fishbowl that holds only male employee names.*

Systematic Sampling

Every X^{th} item or every Y^{th} time period is sampled. This seems easy, but if the total sample is not sorted randomly, it will lead to inaccurate or skewed data. **Example:** *Pulling names out of a fishbowl that holds 100% of employee names, but only using every 5th name.*

Nonprobability Sampling

Subject matter experts make a qualitative judgment and assumptions about a common issue in order to reduce the size of the sample, assuming that the problem is uniform:
- *Convenience sampling: e.g., all patients admitted last week*
- *Purposive sampling: e.g., all patients over 20 who have measles*
- *Quota sampling: e.g., 5% of female breast cancer patients 55–65*

Generally

1. *The sample must be large enough to reliably answer questions about the population and satisfy those who will be scrutinizing.*

2. *The smaller the sample, the less accurate it is likely to be.*

3. *When it's necessary to be very accurate, consult with experts who work in your organization. There are actually people who enjoy working with this stuff who can be resources to the team.*

4. *For efficiency, samples should be small without losing the needed representation. Generally, at least 30 cases or 5% of the population, whichever is greater.[3]*

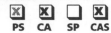

PS   CA   SP   CAS

Scatter Diagram

What A graphic that **displays the relationship** between two variables (e.g., the relationship between an increase in overtime and rise in absenteeism).

Use for Studying the possible relationship between one variable and another:

- Verify a relationship between two variables and point to a possible root cause.

- Monitor and measure results.

When
- To test a theory of the relationship between two variables

- For data analysis - may do several

- To monitor the results of a recently implemented solution

Directions for use

1. From one or more "possible" causes, select two variables to be tested for their relationship to each other.

2. Collect 50 to 100 paired samples of data and record on data sheet.

3. Draw the horizontal X axis (possible cause) and vertical Y axis (problem), noting which represents each variable.

4. Plot the variables on the graph. Indicate repeated values by circling the representative point each time the value is repeated.

Note: The scatter diagram is used to test for "possible" cause and effect relationships. Other data collection will have to <u>prove</u> a causal relationship.

Example

Is there a relationship between overtime (OT) and incidents? Four data sets show four different answers.

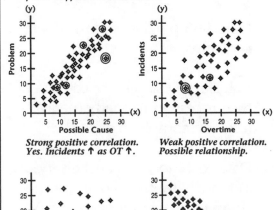

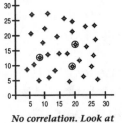
Strong positive correlation. Yes. Incidents ↑ as OT ↑.

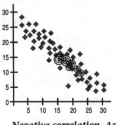
Weak positive correlation. Possible relationship.

No correlation. Look at another probable cause.

Negative correlation. As overtime ↑ incidents ↓.

Interpretation

1. **Strong positive correlation** – An increase in (x) may affect the results of (y). If (x) can be controlled, so might the outcomes of (y).

2. **Weak (possible) positive correlation** – A possible relationship, but there may be several causes or another stronger relationship (another "possible" root cause may be in control).

3. **No correlation** – There is no evidence that results of (y) are related to or are influenced by this variable. Additional data collection is not likely to verify this as a **cause** and is, therefore, not warranted.

4. **Negative correlation** – There is no evidence to support this as a possible root cause (but still important information). As OT rises, incidents go down.

PS CA SP CAS

Statistical Process Control & Normal Variation

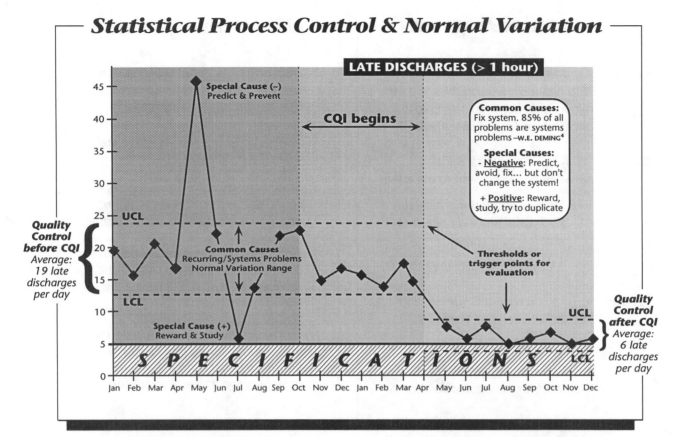

LATE DISCHARGES (> 1 hour)

CQI begins

Common Causes:
Fix system. 85% of all problems are systems problems –W.E. DEMING[4]

Special Causes:
- **Negative**: Predict, avoid, fix... but don't change the system!

+ **Positive**: Reward, study, try to duplicate

Special Cause (–)
Predict & Prevent

UCL

Quality Control before CQI
Average: 19 late discharges per day

Common Causes
Recurring/Systems Problems
Normal Variation Range

LCL

Special Cause (+)
Reward & Study

Thresholds or trigger points for evaluation

UCL

Quality Control after CQI
Average: 6 late discharges per day

LCL

S P E C I F I C A T I O N S

Jan Feb Mar Apr May Jun Jul Aug Sep Oct Nov Dec Jan Feb Mar Apr May Jun Jul Aug Sep Oct Nov Dec

---

Specifications
(a.k.a: Standards, indicators, goals, targets, wishes)

- Indicates the level of **performance you need** and **want**.

- Based on what is required by **employees**, the **customer**, and the **process** itself.

- Data collection and analysis should indicate if the process is **performing as it should**.

- **Example**: Zero incidents of lost dentures. Zero dollars paid.

Control Limits
(a.k.a: Norms, thresholds, normal range of variation)

- Indicates how the process **usually performs.**

- **Calculated** using historical data of the process and a mathematical formula (consult an expert).

- Data collection and analysis should indicate if **process** is doing **something unusual** (out of control?).

- **Example**: Decrease incidents of lost dentures and dollars paid by a minimum of 2% by date.

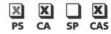

PS CA SP CAS

Success Plan

What *A way to **plan for action**. It's an interactive and enjoyable tool that allows participants to be negative and still achieve positive results.*

Use for *Identifying outcomes and action steps to make any change:*
- *Achieve a **goal**.*
- *Make an improvement.*
- ***Solve** a problem.*
- ***Prevent** a problem.*

When
- ***Quick problem solutions** or prevention steps are needed.*
- *Expected results need to be identified for an action plan.*
- ***Group energy is low** or already negative... put it to work!*
- ***Innovative ideas** are needed.*

Directions for use
Success Plan

1. **Select a situation you want to change (a goal, an improvement, a problem, or a prevention plan).**

2. **Convene a group who knows and can influence the situation.**

3. **Draw grid (below) on a flipchart.**

4. **Have the group brainstorm ways to fail or make the issue worse!**

5. **After the list is complete, continue using structured brainstorming for another list reversing negative ideas into positive plans:**

- *Turn ideas into positive statements.*
- *Build on positive ideas.*
- *Suggest a completely new idea.*

Example

Staff won't buy into implementing a new process because they're afraid to take the risk

WRITE GOAL RESULT, PROBLEM, OR ISSUE ABOVE

1. How can we increase fear of failure?	2. How can we remove risk as an obstacle?
TO FAIL	**TO SUCCEED**
• Set ridiculous goals.	• Set realistic goals.
• Ignore obstacles, they'll fade away.	• Action plan to remove obstacles.
• Do it all yourself and never delegate.	• Encourage, share ideas, workload, responsibility.
• Have all the answers.	
• Laugh at risk takers.	• Reward risk takers.
• Wing it – do what seems right at the moment.	• Plan how to achieve (process) by when, resource needs.
• Do whatever's easy.	• Ask the experienced, "If you could do it over...?"

Combination
Success + Action Plan

WRITE GOAL RESULT, PROBLEM, OR ISSUE ABOVE

TO FAIL	WHAT/OBJECTIVE	HOW
	TO SUCCEED	**ACTION**
	Use ideas from the SUCCEED column to "step" into the first two columns of an action plan:	
Do whatever's easy	Ask the experienced, "If you could do it over again, what would you do differently?"	Research: Who's done this and done it well.
		Create a standard interview form.
		Assign contact calls to team members and progress report date.

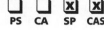

PS   CA   SP   CAS

Task List

What   A simple list, in process analysis, it is often used to generate a list of data (to collect) that will help analyze and confirm the root cause.

Use for   Generating a list of:
- Problems/processes to improve
- Data to collect
- Possible solutions
- Indicators to monitor

How
- Referencing a fishbone, flowchart, or other work, use consensus to highlight the most significant and likely "possible" root causes.
- List data that will confirm.
- Determine if the data are available, and if not, where they can be found and how they will be collected.

Task list hints

1. What data do we need to analyze?	2. Where is it? Will we borrow data or collect?	3. How will data be collected? Survey, Observation Sampling, Checksheet?
What data will help you verify that the "perceived" root cause is, in fact, the true root cause of the problem?	• Computer • Log books • Outcome studies • Medical record • Department records • Payroll • If you don't know where it's located in your organization… find out fast!	• **Survey** —Written —Phone —Interview • **Observation** or experiential • **Sampling** — _Random_ - Most common. By pure chance. — _Stratified_ - By age, gender, hair color, etc. — _Systematic_ - Every Xth occurrence — _Combination_ - Above methods can be combined • **Checksheet** —Simple tabulation —Visual —Matrix —Symbol

Example 1

1. What data do we need to analyze?	2. Where is it? Will we borrow data or collect?	3. How will data be collected? Survey, Observation Sampling, Checksheet?
Problem: Late discharges are slowing the patient flow and backing up patients in ICU and the ED.		
Late discharges per day	On nursing units. Collect.	Observation and checksheet
Why patients remain in room postdischarge	Patients can provide this info. Collect.	Survey: written, interview, or both
What would motivate them to go home?	Patients, physicians, nursing staff. Collect.	Survey: written, oral, or both
Is it occurring on all nursing units?	In the task force records. Borrow.	NA

Example 2

1. What data do we need to analyze?	2. Where is it? Will we borrow data or collect?	3. How will data be collected? Survey, Observation Sampling, Checksheet?
A team is working on improving the clinical path for open heart surgery (OHS) patients.		
Number of OHS patients: With cardiac rehab (CR), without CR, or partial	Raw data are on patient's medical record. Collect.	Tally and display on a scatter diagram.
Number of readmissions	To be found in unit log books	Tally and display on a checksheet.
Reasons for readmissions	Utilization review has been tracking this info for months.	Pareto diagram root causes of readmit

PS   CA   SP   CAS

Action Meeting Minutes

Conclusions:

Recommendations:

Objective What are the expected results?	Action How will results be accomplished? Specifically, what steps will be taken? How will results be measured?	Resources Labor, supply, and equipment costs	• Completion Date (When) • Responsible Person (Who)

Continues

Action Meeting Minutes *(continued)*

page _____ of _____

Objective What are the expected results?	Action How will results be accomplished? Specifically, what steps will be taken? How will results be measured?	Resources Labor, supply, and equipment costs	• Completion Date (When) • Responsible Person (Who)

Action Planning Form

Objective What are the expected results?	Action <u>How</u> will results be accomplished? Specifically, what steps will be taken?	Resources needed & their cost (Labor, supplies, equipment)	Indicator How will results be measured?	• Completion Date (When) • Responsible Person (Who)

Activity Time Log
Capturing workload by outcome, process, and time

Function, task, or intervention	**Staff Member Instructions:** Each time a task/activity is performed (1) write in the next open box how many minutes it took to complete (2) initial

Calculating Standards
Using Retrospective Classification Data

Department or Service Line Modalities	Modalities Completed & Charged	Required Hours per Modality*	Staff Hours Required
_____	_____ X _____		= _____
_____	_____ X _____		= _____
_____	_____ X _____		= _____
_____	_____ X _____		= _____
_____	_____ X _____		= _____
_____	_____ X _____		= _____
Totals			

* *Hours are gathered from logging or classification data and reflect only direct, hands-on care. Fixed hours (manager, clerks) and nonproductive hours (sick, vacation, etc.) are not included at this point.*

Total Staff Hrs Required ÷ Total Period Modalities = Average Required Labor Hours per Modality Based on Acuity *and* Volume

_____ ÷ _____ = _____

Cost-Benefit Analysis

PROPOSED SOLUTION OR OPTION   **ANALYSIS PERIOD**

TANGIBLE COSTS	DOLLAR VALUE	TANGIBLE BENEFITS	DOLLAR VALUE
•	$ -----------	•	$ -----------
•	$ -----------	•	$ -----------
•	$ -----------	•	$ -----------
•	$ -----------	•	$ -----------
•	$ -----------	•	$ -----------
•	$ -----------	•	$ -----------
•	$ -----------	•	$ -----------
•	$ -----------	•	$ -----------
• **Total Costs**	$ -----------	• **Total Benefits**	$ -----------

INTANGIBLE COSTS	**INTANGIBLE BENEFITS**
•	•
•	•
•	•
•	•

$$\text{Cost Benefit Ratio} = \frac{\text{Benefits} \; (\qquad)}{\text{Costs} \; (\qquad)} = \underline{\qquad}$$

Criteria Grid*

EVALUATION CRITERIA

ISSUE TO PRIORITIZE

*Also commonly known as **Selection Grid**, **Decision Matrix**, and **Prioritization Matrix***

Mission & Vision	Strategic Priorities/Goals	Performance Improvement Priorities/Goals	Annual Measures	Cross-Functional Projects

Deploying Mission, Vision, and Priorities

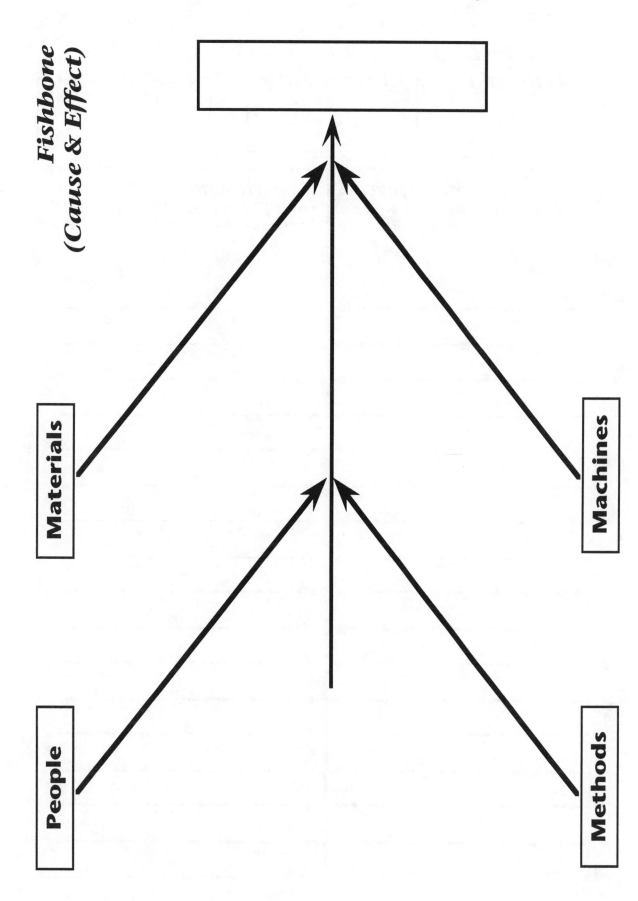

Fishbone (Cause & Effect)

Force Field Analysis

Current State	Goal/Solution

Driving forces
existing circumstances that will help achieve desired state

Resisting forces
existing forces (obstacles) keeping us from achieving our goal

Care or Service Outcome Indicators
Care (clinical and satisfaction) or service results

Performance or Process Indicators
Recommended process and employee responsibilities

Financial Indicators
Necessary or avoidable cost

Strategic Priority: _____

Performance Improvement Priority: _____

Indicator Development Worksheet

Care or Service Outcome Indicators
Care (clinical and satisfaction) or service results

Performance or Process Indicators
Recommended process and employee responsibilities

Financial Indicators
Necessary or avoidable cost

Indicator Assessment Plan

Issue Clarification

1. Today's reality
What is happening?
List and prioritize the core
issue for the team to study.

2. Prioritized critical or core issue:

Broad Issue:

3. Consequence/result
Is this important?
List and prioritize the
ramifications of this issue and
why it's worthwhile to work on.

4. Improvement goal
A success would be:
List and prioritize how you'd
know the problem was fixed
or process was improved.

Sub-Issues:

Outcome & Process Indicators

Outcome or result • The "right" thing to do • Standard of care/service •	• Process or procedure • The "right" way to do it • Standard of performance
What outcome or result are we seeking (delighted customers, saved lives, improved quality of life)? What end or purpose are we targeting?	What process, method, or procedure will we follow to ensure achievement of those outcomes (results) on a routine and predictable basis?

PERSONAL WORK LOG ANALYSIS

During the next two weeks, please keep a log of how you spend your time at work. In particular, log the things that take up big chunks of your time (staffing, crisis management, disciplining employees, etc.). Answer the questions for each activity, add your total time consumed, and bring this with you to the workshop.

WHAT I DID/ACTIVITY	HOW MUCH OF MY TIME WAS CONSUMED?	WAS IT THE RIGHT THING TO DO?	DID I DO IT THE RIGHT WAY? WAS THE BEST PROCESS USED?

Project Analysis

1. Strategic goal the project addresses _____
_____

2. Specific process to be improved _____
_____

3. Customer(s) to be served _____ Internal _____ External _____

4. Disciplines/functions involved in or affected by improvement _____
_____
_____

5. This effort should improve _____

6. This process is important to work on now because _____
_____
_____

7. How will results be measured _____
_____
_____

8. _____ is the sponsor and representative to the PI Council.

9. Start date _____ Project Team is _____
Progress check dates _____ Finish date is _____
Leader _____ Facilitator _____ (Membership list attached)

10. Constraints/parameters, instructions to the team from the PI Council _____
_____
_____
_____

11. Estimated # of labor hours/team hours for the project _____
Expected return on investment (attach Cost-Benefit Analysis) _____
_____

12. Reviewed/approved by PI Council _____ Date _____

Project Checklist

***After a project or issue is selected and clarified, compare it
to this checklist to ensure getting off on the right foot.***

❑ *Team **agrees** on the **project** and can clearly describe in a sentence or
two (1) the issue, (2) why it needs to be addressed, and (3) the desired improvement goal.*

❑ *Both the team members and management believe the project and
its potential payoff is **achievable** and **worth** the team's time.*

❑ *The project (or prioritized sub-issue) is **narrow** enough to maintain
the focus of the group.*

❑ *There is **support for change** and **improvement** related to the
project issues (from managers, employees, customers).*

❑ *The project is related (directly or indirectly) to an important **cross-
functional issue.***

❑ *The process is **repetitive**, is **not in transition,** and is not being
studied by another group.*

❑ *Current process, if one exists, is **stable** and **clearly defined** (including the start and end points).*

❑ ***Start-up projects:** Select an issue that (1) is important but uncomplicated enough to be resolved quickly, (2) showcases the value
of CQI, and (3) involves those who will buy in, apply what they've
learned, and champion the effort.*

Resource Utilization Report Card

Modality Description or Patient Class Level	Sunday	Monday	Tuesday	Wednesday	Thursday	Friday	Saturday	Sunday	Monday	Tuesday	Wednesday	Thursday	Friday	Saturday	Total Modalities or Patient Days	Hours per Modality (HPM) or Patient Day (HPPD)	Total Classified (Weighted & Acuity Required) Hours
	+	+	+	+	+	+	+	+	+	+	+	+	+	=	X	=	
TOTALS																	

A. Total pay period patient days or modalities   _____

B. Total weighted required hours (from above)   _____

C. Total hours actually provided (source: payroll, Productivity and Acuity Report, or a simple manual count of actual staffed hours)   _____

D. Hours per patient day or modality:
  1) **Budget** (the standard remains constant throughout fiscal year)   _____
  2) **Classified** (weighted and acuity required) [B ÷ A]   _____
  3) **Actual** staffed hours provided [C ÷ A]   _____

E. Productivity Indexes (using figures from D.1, D.2, and D.3 for formulas)

  1) Actual staffed hours provided to budgeted hours: $\dfrac{\text{Hours Provided}}{\text{Hours Budgeted}}$ or $\dfrac{\text{D.3}}{\text{D.1}}$ _____

  2) Actual staffed hours provided to classified hours: $\dfrac{\text{Hours Provided}}{\text{Hours Required}}$ or $\dfrac{\text{D.3}}{\text{D.2}}$ _____

REWARD & RECOGNIZE

FREEBIES... OR VERY CLOSE *Managers are free to administer as desired* REWARDS UNDER $50 *Managers can award with approval of direct supervisor* REWARDS OVER $50 *Criteria based – administrative or committee approval required*	IS THE BRAINSTORMED REWARD A FREEBIE, OVER $50, OR UNDER $50?
1.	1.
2.	2.
3.	3.
4.	4.
5.	5.
6.	6.
7.	7.
8.	8.
9.	9.
10.	10.
11.	11.
12.	12.
13.	13.
14.	14.
15.	15.

SPECIFICALLY, WHEN SHOULD WE USE FREEBIES, UNDER $50, AND OVER $50 TO PRAISE EFFORTS?

Skills Checklist
for Facilitators & Team Leaders

Facilitator* Competencies	Not Met	Met	Exceeded	Improvement Ideas
TOPIC INTRODUCTION				
• Presents crisp opening (clear agenda/objectives)	___	___	___	_____
• Gives background & connecting information	___	___	___	_____
• Is enthusiastic, generates positive energy	___	___	___	_____
GROUP INVOLVEMENT				
• Asks effective questions, listens, and reflects back to group when appropriate	___	___	___	_____
• Uses examples to illustrate points and help cement concepts/tools	___	___	___	_____
• Uses activities to guide group to objectives	___	___	___	_____
• Leads group discussions and reinforces their participation (acknowledges contributions by flipcharting key points, paraphrasing, restating, summarizing, and nonverbal gesturing)	___	___	___	
SMOOTH TRANSITION				
• Paces group discussions and activities within time constraints	___	___	___	_____
• Uses transitions for closure and linkages to next topic or point	___	___	___	_____
• Clarifies and summarizes key learning points	___	___	___	_____
MISCELLANEOUS				
• Takes care of the group—stays tuned in, explores and responds to the groups' needs	___	___	___	_____
• Plans/prepares learning objectives, activities, presentation format, and audiovisuals	___	___	___	_____
• Revises agenda as necessary	___	___	___	_____

Success Planning

WRITE GOAL RESULT, PROBLEM, <u>OR</u> ISSUE ABOVE

What can be done to ensure failure	*What can be done to ensure success*

Success + Action Plan

WRITE GOAL RESULT, PROBLEM, OR ISSUE ABOVE

What can we do to ensure failure?	*What can we do to ensure success?*	*How? What process should we follow?*

Task List for Data

What data do we need to analyze?	*Where is it? Will we borrow data or collect it?*	*How will we collect the data?* *Survey, Sampling, Computer, Logs, Observation, Checksheet?*

TEAM BINGO

I've led a team using CQI methods _____	I can't facilitate without a flipchart _____	I'm interested in group dynamics _____	I've been on a dysfunctional team _____	I know how questions help team leaders _____
I'm nervous when I have to facilitate _____	I know an icebreaker I can share _____	QI methods are used in my dept. _____	I am empowered in my work _____	We use QI in all of our org. meetings _____
I've been able to involve physicians _____	I've been on a clinical pathway team _____	**Free**	I'm a process improvement team member _____	We often use cost-benefit analysis _____
I can name 3 of my internal customers _____	I've used QI techniques with my family _____	I didn't buy this QI stuff at first _____	I believe mistakes can be treasures _____	I like flowcharting _____
Our vision is clear and well known by all _____	I've helped implement a team solution _____	I've already delivered QI training _____	I know a resource to recommend _____	I periodically rush to solution _____

Directions: Walk around the room, meet your colleagues, and ask of they'll sign in one (only one) of your boxes. Instead of a line, the "Bingo" will be a **full card** or the number of people in the room. Every box will have to be signed by a different person in the room.

Notes

1. Joint Commission on Accreditation of Healthcare Organizations, *Accreditation Manual for Hospitals: Volume II* (Oakbrook Terrace, IL: 1994), 18.

2. Joint Commission on Accreditation of Healthcare Organizations, *Accreditation Manual for Hospitals* (OakbrookTerrace, IL: 1996), 102.

3. Joint Commission, *Accreditation Manual for Hospitals* (1994),18.

4. W.E. Deming, *Out of Crisis* (Cambridge, MA: Center for Advanced Engineering Study, Massachusetts Institute of Technology, 1986).

Recommended Reading

Brassard, M. 1989. *Memory Jogger Plus+.* Methuen, MA: Goal/QPC.

Brassard, M., and D. Ritter. 1994. *The Memory Jogger.* Methuen, MA: Goal/QPC.

Coffey, R. et al., Winter 1995. Extending the application of critical path methods. *Quality Management in Health Care.* 14–29.

Kern, J.P. January 1993. Toward total quality marketing. *Quality Progress.* 39–42.

Luttman, R. et al., Winter 1995. Using PERT/CPM to design and improve clinical processes. *Quality Management in Health Care.* 1–12.

WHEN IN DOUBT STAY WITH THE GROUP

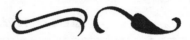

WHEN THE GROUP STARTS TALKING TO EACH OTHER, INSTEAD OF YOU, YOU'RE FACILITATING

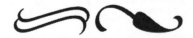

TRUST THE GROUP

Facilitator Survival Guide

- **BRING OUT THE BEST IN YOUR TEAM**

- **HELP IMPROVE PERFORMANCE RESULTS**

- **GAIN CONFIDENCE IN YOUR ABILITY TO FACILITATE AND WORK A GROUP**

INTRODUCTION

If you've ever been up in front of a team—feeling responsible and accountable for results—you already understand the need for this guide, and you already know how challenging it is to facilitate.

Just as continuous quality improvement (CQI) tools and scientific method became indispensable to managers, facilitation skills will be the next "must-have" skill for executives, managers, work-team leaders, committee chairs, and task force leaders. Personally, you may be in a leadership position, but you're also part of a team. Do you like to be given mandates and lists of things to do, without the opportunity to provide input? Or do you prefer to be involved in decisions and have a say in how things are done? Most people from line employees through the chief executive officer (CEO) think they have something of value to contribute... and they're right! Facilitation skills furnish valuable contributors with an opportunity to share in problem solving and decision making about the things they know best... their work.

Initially, team leaders are consumed with mastering the tools in the tool-box. Clearly, that is the right choice because using the tools will force the leader into a facilitating style. When tools are used, the leader is forced to ask questions, forced to open up the topic to discussion, and forced to follow the thoughts of the group. Without process management tools, it is easy to fall back on lecturing, making all the decisions, and trying to come up with all the answers. There are few among us who have all the answers, and there are mountains of evidence to demonstrate the value of synergy—that a group of bright, talented people can come up with a better output than the best of the individual members combined.

It's the job of facilitators to bring out the best in a team. It's their choice of tools, their questions, their probing, their knowing when the group is on a tangent—or moving toward consensus—that can make a difference. It is rewarding and inspiring work, but it is also challenging, and sometimes frightening, and that's why this guide was created.

FACILITATOR SURVIVAL GUIDE
CONTENTS

PREPARE FOR FACILITATION

KNOWLEDGE

Materials: Know what you need and keep a list.
Participants: Know who they are and what their agendas are.
Program structure
Group dynamics: Know when to respond, draw out, or move on.
Videotapes and equipment
Learning psychology
  • defensive/resistant
  • adult learning
Goals and direction
Empathy: How it feels to be a participant

WISDOM

One thought-provoking or discussion-producing question is worth 10,000 words.
When in doubt, stay with the group (instead of your notes, write notes on flipchart).
Closure: seek opportunities to close discussion when 80% of issues are out.
Whenever possible, pick consensus over voting.
Soliciting participation is better than calling on someone. If they're not participating, privately ask them why.
Be aware of seating and the impact of moving participants around the room.
Tell group (1) what you're going to tell them, (2) then tell them, (3) then tell them what you told them.

DEVELOP SKILLS

Clear communication:
  • Listening
  • Questioning
  • Clarifying
  • Summarizing
  • Restating
  • Paraphrasing
Humor
Courage
Enthusiasm
Flexibility
Thinking on one's feet
Keeping cool and focused under pressure
Maximize group dynamics.
Can play devil's advocate
Sensitive to group
Expect the unexpected.
Planning
Meeting management and control
Draw out a discovery rather than trying to convince.
Manage flipcharts.
Believe in program.
Be a role model.
Share goals, reiterate.
Ready and prepared for potential *"so what"*?
Able to bring a group out and close for transition
Use bullets in your speech.
Breaks: Say <u>when</u> to return
Flipchart video questions
Techniques for motivating the group to read pre-reading:
  • Refer to it.
  • Let group summarize.
  • Use reinforcement.
  • Give class time to read.
  • Fill them in yourself.
Write big and clear. Use colors and lined pads.
Practice • Practice • Practice

GENERAL TIPS

Be prepared.
Use flipcharts (FC) and hang them for reference. Check for bleeding on walls. Let partner scribe for you. Cap markers. Write pencil notes.
Tab/flag FCs for quick access.
Clip corresponding book pages.
Write page numbers on FCs.
To keep discussion going, draw some things from book on FC to keep eyes and attention with the group.
Use the whole room. Walk and remove physical barriers.
Reflect questions—throw them back to the group rather than answer yourself.
Don't try to be the expert.
Review schedule plans.
Be available for homework help.
Tell group about restrooms, breaks, lunch, and general housekeeping details.
Recapture energy and participation by acknowledging it:
  • Take a break.
  • Talk about it.
  • Make activity more active.
  • Break into groups.
Place a clock in front of you.
Prepare video set-up ahead.
Using words like *we* and *us* (vs. *you* and *I*) help make a facilitator part of the group.
Facilitate and draw out existing knowledge and discoveries rather than teach or lecture. Even in lecturettes, ask yourself: Is there any way I can get this from the group?
Check in with the group occasionally: How are we doing?
If you err, acknowledge it, fix it, and move on. Set a tone that it's okay to make a mistake.

ROLES & RESPONSIBILITIES: FACILITATOR

Responsible for helping teams (cross-functional, task force, and natural work teams) effectively pursue the process of improving performance and sustaining the improvement over time. Facilitators educate and coach team leaders in group dynamics and process skills that are necessary for problem solving, process improvement (redesign), and process design (reengineering). **The concentration is on "how," the action, the process.**

Specific responsibilities:

1. Understands, supports, and feels ownership for the team's goals
2. Remains neutral to the subject, but passionate about the process
3. Listens and acknowledges, without judgment (by repeating, writing on a flipchart, nodding, etc.) all input from team
4. Is able to focus on both the task and the team dynamics concurrently
5. Understands and feels comfortable with productive conflict, knowing when and how to mediate and help resolve, bring to closure, or transition
6. Trusts and builds trust among members
7. Communicates assertively, openly, and honestly
8. Is knowledgeable of available resources, uses them as needed, and communicates their availability to the team
9. Continually helps the team work toward and achieve consensus (i.e., negotiated general agreement, without pressure or threat) and closure so they can move to the next step of their work
10. Solicits opinions, clarifies and blends different ideas, and checks for/summarizes consensus. Seeks input from all members, ensuring equal participation
11. Ensures that documentation is created, maintained, and distributed
12. Provides feedback to and teaches team leaders about the use of tools and group process technique
13. Helps the team assess its effectiveness and plan for improvement
14. Conducts team leader training and coaches assigned leaders ongoing; helping plan, suggesting useful tools, assessing and giving feedback on their leadership skills
15. Communicates with quality council as needed and appropriate
16. Helps organize and assign internal consulting or facilitating, as necessary

Needs to know:

1. Quality management theory and concepts
2. Problem solving/process improvement tools and skills (from the toolbox)
3. Group process skills and the fundamentals of how groups behave

(continues)

ROLES & RESPONSIBILITIES: FACILITATOR

(CONTINUED)

4. How to handle conflict and interventions
5. Hands-on experience of how adult learners learn
6. How to be comfortable in front of a group... even under pressure

Desirable characteristics or achievements:

1. Rating in the top 10% of their peer group in performance appraisals

2. Track record of credibility and perceived as such by peers

3. Resilience and nondefensiveness when challenged or confronted

4. Commitment to modeling high standards of personal integrity and quality work

5. Bright future and potential for growth within the organization

6. Creative optimism and belief that improvement is possible

7. Flexibility—comfortable with rapid changes of direction

8. Interest in and motivation to take on this role

9. Ability to maintain sense of humor

10. Good people skills; likes people and is likable

11. High tolerance for ambiguity and conflict

12. Self-confidence but not arrogance

13. High energy level/stamina

14. Humility—willingness to make mistakes and learn from them

15. Understanding of and ability to help others see the big picture

16. Ability to say a lot in a few words and get a message across

17. Street smart about office politics

18. Willingness to share center stage and support others' growth in the process

19. Knowledge of the techniques yet willing to work toward continued improvement

20. Good organizational skills; well organized

**FACILITATOR
SELECTION
&
DEVELOPMENT**

FLOWCHART

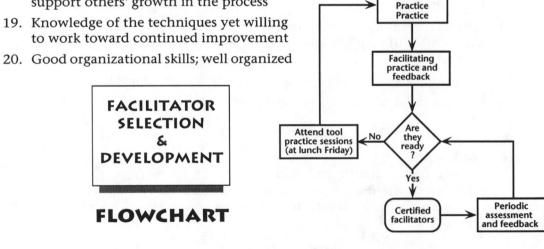

ROLES & RESPONSIBILITIES: TEAM LEADER

Responsible for moving teams (cross-functional, task force, and natural work teams) through the actual process of improving performance and sustaining the improvement over time. Team leaders use group dynamics and process skills for problem solving, process improvement (redesign), and process design (reengineering). **Concentration is on "what," the goal, the outcome.**

Specific responsibilities:
1. Organizes, arranges, and leads team meetings and uses meeting management skills and pacing to ensure a productive output
2. Owns and supports the team's goals, restating as needed to keep the group focused
3. Remains neutral to the subject (if there is no facilitator) and true to the process
4. Listens and acknowledges (repeats, writes on a flipchart, etc.) all input from team
5. Is able to focus on both the task and the team dynamics concurrently
6. Understands and feels comfortable with productive conflict, knowing when and how to mediate and help resolve, bring to closure, or transition
7. Trusts and builds trust among members by being open, honest, fair, and consistent
8. Communicates assertively, openly, and honestly, providing appropriate and adequate information to the team. Is respectful to the organization and team members
9. Is knowledgeable of available resources (including other teams), uses them as needed, and communicates their availability to the team
10. Continually helps the team work toward and achieve consensus (i.e., negotiated general agreement, without pressure or threat) and closure
11. Solicits opinions, clarifies and blends different ideas, and checks for/summarizes consensus. Seeks input from all members, ensuring equal participation
12. Creates, maintains, and distributes documentation tracking and measuring progress
13. Helps team members assess their effectiveness and plan for improvement, creating an atmosphere of growth, using positive improvement strategies, recognition, reward
14. Communicates with superiors to apprise them of the team's progress
15. Accepts responsibility for team performance, effectiveness, and productivity

Needs to know:
1. Problem solving/process improvement theory, concepts, tools, and skills
2. Team leader, group process, and meeting management skills
3. How to handle conflict and interventions
4. As much about the process being studied as possible

Desirable characteristics or achievements:
1. Track record of credibility and is perceived as such by peers
2. Good people skills—likes people and is likable; trusts and is trusted
3. Commitment to high standards of personal integrity and quality work
4. Positive outlook, with creative optimism and belief that improvement is possible
5. Able to bring out the best in others, yet willing to share center stage and recognition
6. Flexibility—comfort with rapid changes of direction, ambiguity, and conflict
7. Resilience and nondefensiveness when challenged or confronted
8. Humility—willingness to make and learn from mistakes (and maintain sense of humor)
9. Understanding of and ability to help others see the big picture
10. Ability to say a lot in a few words and get a message across
11. Interest in and motivation to take on this role and lead a team
12. Knowledge of the organization and how it works
13. Good organizational skills; well organized
14. Loyal—commitment to the organization and its long-term success

ROLES & RESPONSIBILITIES: TEAM MEMBER

Responsible for sharing their expert knowledge of the topic at hand. As process owners, they know better than anyone else what is wrong with the process, the early warning signs of trouble, how to fix the problem, and how to prevent it from occurring again.

Specific responsibilities:
1. Participates in setting and adheres to the team's Ground Rules
2. Helps define, action plan, and support the team's goals
3. Attends all meetings and participates in discussions, tools, and decision activities
4. Makes every effort to look at the process from others' vantage points
5. Shares information from their perspective and listens to others' input
6. Completes responsibilities that are assigned between meetings
7. Trusts and builds trust among members
8. Communicates assertively, openly, and honestly
9. Helps create and maintain reports that track and measure progress
10. May periodically be assigned the role of recorder, time keeper, or on-tracker
11. Helps the team assess their effectiveness and plan for improvement
12. Communicates with superiors to apprise them of team progress
13. Helps implement solutions and recommendations and helps monitor results

Needs to know:
1. How the process works
2. Team meeting ground rules
3. Their team member responsibilities

Desirable characteristics or achievements:
1. Track record of credibility and is perceived as such by peers
2. Good people skills—likes people and is likable, trusts and is trusted
3. Commitment to high standards of personal integrity and quality work
4. Positive outlook, with creative optimism and belief that improvement is possible
5. Willingness to share center stage and recognition. Support of others' growth in the process
6. Flexibility—comfort with rapid changes of direction, ambiguity, and conflict
7. Ability to maintain sense of humor
8. Resilience and nondefensiveness when challenged or confronted
9. Humility—willingness to make mistakes and learn from them
10. Understanding of and ability to help others see the big picture
11. Ability to say a lot in a few words and get a message across
12. Interest in and motivation to take on this role
13. Knowledge of the techniques but willingness to work toward continuous improvement
14. Good organizational skills; well organized

CONQUERING FEAR OF THE GROUP

Public speaking ranks <u>first</u> on David Wallechinsky's[1] list of the *"10 Worst Fears in the U.S.,"* ahead of death (7), sickness (6), and financial problems (4). Like any other fear, the more you face it, and do it, the less terrifying it becomes. Here are some other tips:

1. To be authentic and convincing, be a **subject matter expert** if you're teaching or a **group process skills expert** if you're facilitating.

2. **Practice**. Practice. Practice—with a public speaking group or any friendly group that will give you useful, improvement-focused feedback or even a videotape. Mentally rehearse answers to tough questions. If you don't know the answer, admit it, ask the group if they know, and assure them you'll find out and let them know.

3. Take the focus off of yourself by **involving the group**. Open with a question; start a discussion or an icebreaker activity.

4. **Learn participants' names** and use them.[2] Tent cards or stick-on name badges accelerate the memorization process. (Caution: If you move participants to another seat for an activity, ask them to move their tent cards also.)

5. **Physical releases**: Arrive rested. Deep breathe. Stretch. Walk. Meditate. Pass candy.

6. Use **humor**, and it doesn't have to be a joke. One participant who suddenly got very tongue-tied said, "If I could talk, here's what I'd say." Everyone laughed, he caught his breath, and he was back on track.

7. Use **eye contact** to establish rapport[3] and to read the group for nonverbal feedback.

8. Exhibit your **advance preparation**[4] (handouts, overheads, knowledge, background information). Enthusiasm is contagious. Don't be afraid to let yours show.

9. **Be yourself**. There's a reason you were asked to teach/facilitate. Believe in yourself.

10. **Avoid reading**. In fact, if you can avoid it, don't even write out what you're going to say because your eyes will lock in and you'll end up reading. Write out key points on a flip chart (you can pencil in some notes or write on a removable note) or an outline. If you must write out what you want to say, highlight key points in a highlighter pen.

11. **Advance preparation**: (1) Identify purpose and session objectives and prepare a session that will meet the objectives and the needs of your customers. (2) Seek information on the group, potential problems, and dress. (3) Check out equipment, facilities, and room setup for comfort, practicality, and workability.

12. Start the session by asking the group for their "**burning issue**," the one thing they would (realistically) like resolved or addressed by the end of the session. Participants will decide in the first few minutes whether or not the session is worthwhile. If you focus on what is important to them, you'll draw in their interest, attention, and enthusiasm.

13. Overview session **objectives**, conduct the session, and recap what was accomplished.

14. **Meet participants** in advance (by phone prior to session or by greeting as they arrive).

15. With a group of peers, list **worst fears**, and brainstorm some possible solutions.

16. If nothing works, and you're still in a panic, don't despair; nervous energy will keep you sharp, and audiences usually empathize and support a nervous speaker.

CHARACTERS YOU'LL MEET WHEN FACILITATING
...AND HOW TO SURVIVE THEM!

The know-it-all or overbearing participant
If someone is using his or her external authority, expertise, or seniority to influence the group, your job is to remind everyone of their equality on the team. Ask experts to share information so everyone is at an equal knowledge level. Ask for cooperation and patience and stay focused on the tools and the process. Use them to summarize.

The arguer
Relax and <u>do</u> <u>not</u> argue back. Ask questions to reflect the issue back to the group, clarify the issue and areas of agreement, and defuse the discussion. Let the team members debate the issue.

The shy person
Brainstorm. Wallstorm. Have a smaller meeting where discussion is easier. Ask some simple, no-risk questions to pull shy members into the discussion. Use both verbal (I see, hmmm, okay) and nonverbal (smile, nod, eye contact) signals to draw the person in. Use paraphrasing or probing questions to draw out more participation.

The grudge-bearer
Start with a ground rule: no rehashing. Give the group a predetermined amount of time to vent (flipchart their output). Once documented, the grudge-bearer will have an easier time letting go.

The talker and monopolizer
Use the tools… use the tools… use the tools. Forcing responses in an organized fashion brings out the shy people and restricts the talkers. Avoid eye contact. Talk to monopolizer outside of the meeting. Invite others' ideas. If necessary, create a ground rule to address. Ask him or her to help you get others involved. Ask the team to agree on and reinforce limits and stay focused in discussions.

The latecomer
Close the door and start on time no matter who is there. Put the most important agenda items first, especially those of interest to the latecomers. Keep a constant meeting time. Try peer pressure or speaking privately to offenders.

The giver of bad or incomplete ideas
There's no such thing as a bad idea. Judging will only get you in trouble. So no judging! Encourage speaker to tell more about his or her idea. Ask questions to clarify. Restate in a more concise form, if necessary, without changing the meaning. Check with the person for agreement, and thank him or her for the input.

The deferrer who asks, "What's your opinion?"
Beware of this trap as it forces you into an "expert" or "judging" role, and the group will begin to defer to you routinely. Make your neutrality clear to the group, offering opinions only about the process. Throw the question back to the group, "Who has some information on this?" Or ask clarifying questions.

The procrastinator
Use *Action Minutes* to document <u>what</u>'s to be done, <u>how</u> it will be accomplished, <u>who</u> is responsible, and the <u>target</u> <u>date</u> for completion. Give or send them to members quickly so they have minutes *and* a reminder of their homework assignment.

(continues)

CHARACTERS YOU'LL MEET...

The put-down attacker (or the ignorer) a.k.a. Sender of verbal hits and memo missiles

Possible ground rules: no put-downs. All ideas will be given respect and equal consideration. Treat the idea as you would any other that you're receiving. Remind the group of the "no judging" rule. Thank the person for his or her input. Introduce the *Quarter Pot* which requires people to pay $.25 when they make a disparaging remark about anyone in the group or his or her ideas. Explain to the group the negative repercussions and damaging effects of this behavior.

The tangent taker (a.k.a. digressor)

Use a written agenda with time estimates. Use a flipchart and title it. Comment, "We're off the topic," or "Didn't we just reach consensus on that?" (and point to the flip chart that documents that agreement). Refocus by restating purpose, summarizing what's been accomplished, and continue with the tool you were using. Accept that sometimes you have to digress and resolve an issue before the group can continue. Other times, you can put the issue on a flipchart page titled *Parking Lot* and get back to it at a later time. Quietly pass a bunny or other object to the person who is off on a tangent. It may sound silly but it can be very intimidating and effective.

The emotional team member (who is often at the breaking point)

If you remain calm, so will the participant and the group. Acknowledge his or her feelings as legitimate, "I see you feel strongly about this issue. Can you tell us why your concern is so strong?" Flipchart hisor her concerns. Then discuss with the group or put it in a *Parking Lot* for later attention. Ask if he or she is ready to continue. If not, take a break and talk with him or her to make sure the issues are addressed. This is often a critical turning point for the team, so resist brushing it under the rug. Summarize and refocus the group.

The whisperer of side conversations

A ground rule of "no side conversations" is always a good place to start. Establish eye contact with the offenders and move in their direction. Don't embarrass, but invite their input to the group at large. If necessary, speak to them privately. Emphasize that they are not only distracting others but, more importantly, depriving the group of their valuable input.

The two-faced team member

If a person agrees in the meeting but walks down the hall saying, "I'm not doing that," his or her opinions were not properly aired during the meeting, and true consensus was not achieved. As a facilitator, watch for both verbal and nonverbal signs of consensus, and ask questions or confront people if necessary to bring out and eliminate all dissenting issues. If they are not resolved, they'll seep out, or explode, later on and unravel the work.

The my-department-is-the-only-one-that-matters member

Create a shared vision at the onset, post at all meetings, remind the group as needed, and reward/recognize accordingly. If a member simply can't look at the bigger picture of the process, try having everyone exchange roles for the next meeting. To prepare, ask them to spend at least 1 hour with the person they will be "playing" at the next meeting. This will force them to learn about and understand the other member's point of view.

SOME OTHER COMMON PROBLEMS

The team's going nowhere... fast!	Check on how the project is being handled—what tools are being used, what action has been taken. Review the mission, plan, and problem statement, and compare to the work that's been accomplished. Check team members' data. Ask members what the causes might be and discuss what needs to be done next.
Team members state opinions as if they are facts.	There is simply no substitute for data and the scientific process. Team members will do anything they can to skip this approach, but it's always a mistake. It's those assumptions-as-facts that get us into trouble in the first place and lead us to implement wrong solutions. We must challenge beliefs, ask questions for clarification, demand data to test assumptions, and always ask, "As evidenced by what?"
The team is rushing to solution.	Managers have been rewarded for this behavior for decades, so they'll be hardest to hold back. The got-a-problem-got-a-solution mode is deep-rooted. Your job is to make sure the team members have found the real root cause of the problem (and can back it up with data) before they move to solution finding. Require the use of the scientific process, and share how it has worked for other teams.
Everyone is blaming everyone else.	It's so easy to point the finger, then it's someone else's job to fix it. Actually, when two departments point the finger at each other, they are often *both* right. Ask them to first interview each other as customers and suppliers and set expectations for how they are going to work together to meet each others' needs. Use the scientific process. Ask questions to clarify. Charge a quarter for blaming.
Team members are fighting and not cooperating.	Select team members that have a high probability of getting along. Offer to facilitate an outside-of-team discussion. Remind them of the mutually agreed upon purpose of meeting. Identify areas of agreement and disagreement. Ask "Why?" and resolve each. Have them agree on ground rules for managing future differences. Conduct some cooperation exercises, and remind them that they don't have to like each other to cooperate and work toward a common goal.
A previously "hot" team is now unproductive and absences are growing.	Sometimes teams reach a point where they run out of steam. Don't worry, there are lots of things you can do: send the team on vacation for a few months; split the team into two teams and add new members to both; let volunteers take time off or quit the team and add some fresh talent; let the team work on something fun like rewards and recognition or the annual talent show.
Physicians won't participate.	See next page.

INVOLVING PHYSICIANS

Authorities unanimously agree that physicians should be involved in developing critical paths and practice protocols and parameters. Managers and quality professionals contend that it's torturous to get them involved. (In a Hospitals & Health Networks survey, 42% of the respondents cited "Lack of physician support" as one of the biggest obstacles to pursuing critical paths.)[5] Here are some tips from those who have succeeded:

Respect the physician as a customer

Listen, without judgment, to their concerns, input, questions, and requests for information, services, or materials. Invite them to identify which organization processes, bottlenecks, or pathways they'd like to have studied and then fix them first! After they see positive results, they'll be more inclined to volunteer. Or if physicians have been involved in setting strategic and improvement priorities, work on those related pathways first. Respect and be conservative with their time. Some are even compensated with money, perks, or additional power in the organization.

Information sharing

Physicians, as well as others in the organization, dearly want to know what is going on, so devise a plan to keep them abreast of things:
- *Track their performance against peers and accepted standards.*
- *Give confidential feedback on their efficiency by diagnosis-related group (DRG).*
- *Apprise them of the expected length of stay (LOS).*
- *Provide them with actual LOS data and related costs.*

Get your act together first

Invite physicians to participate only on established, high-performing teams. Since they are not generating revenue at a meeting, it's essential that the meeting be well managed and productive. If they believe their time is well spent, they'll be more likely to return. In the interim, have pathway team members communicate (one on one, published success stories, wall maps, etc.) and market pathways to physicians and natural work teams.

from Brent C. James, M.D....

Several lessons were learned while implementing practice guidelines overseeing ventilator management at LDS Hospital, Salt Lake City:[6]
- *Variation in clinical practice is the villain.*
- *Everyone benefits when variation is reduced.*
- *Physicians respond best to efforts focused on improving patient care quality.*
- *Guidelines are not new news.*
- *Control is a big issue, so LDS gave the clinical team control over the guideline.*
- *Local consensus takes priority over the experts from out of town.*
- *For maximum effectiveness, physicians need credible (clinical data) feedback.*

(continues)

INVOLVING PHYSICIANS

from Scripps Memorial Hospitals...
- *Start with committed physicians who rely on hospital resources (cardiac, ortho).*
- *Select straightforward diagnoses (laminectomy was easier than stroke).*
- *Get patient input to help prioritize process steps and clarify language.*
- *Pathways should be flexible so they can change quickly and continuously as data feedback indicates the need.*
- *Run concurrent pilots (old way/new path) initially to assess and remove flaws.[7]*

from Don Berwick, M.D....
- *Reallocate committee and meeting time rather than just adding another.*
- *Formalize how physicians are involved and their role. Be specific for each issue.*
- *Use data.*
- *Keep your eyes pealed for specialties that may be interested.*
- *Involve physician leaders from the onset.*
- *Connect total quality management (TQM) to guidelines and critical paths.[8]*

Physician education
Include information that will help physicians in their own practices when creating education programs (TQM, CQI, clinical pathways, utilization, productivity) you hope they'll attend. Knowledge obtained can be used for their gain or yours. Reference what is happening at other hospitals.

Set up routine systems for involving physicians
- *Involve them right from the start, from developing standards, to designing the processes to achieve the standards, to measuring outcomes (including identifying mistakes and improper use of resources) and taking action to improve.*
- *Routinely, reaffirm or update standards, pathways, and outcome measures.*
- *If you want physicians to follow your regimen, set up a patient-focused, "auto-pilot" system so it will be easier for them to do it your way.*
- *Maintain a purpose of unflinching dedication to patient quality.*
- *Routinely track and benchmark clinical outcomes and costs resulting from designated practice standards and provide confidential, reliable, timely feedback to physicians.*
- *Ask medical staff to define disciplinary measures and criteria for use.*
- *Link pathways to standing physician orders, outcome measures, documentation systems, and communication networks.*

Ensure support from support services
If you're asking physicians to follow your "best" critical path, make sure its achievable and supported by all ancillary, clinical, and support services. The more available the organization is at providing support and guidance (especially to physicians with irregular utilization patterns), the more connected the physician will feel to the organization and its goals.

FACILITATING INTERVENTIONS

Facilitators are responsible for drawing out the expert knowledge of the team members, without manipulating or judging their output. Here are some questions or phrases you can use if you find yourself at a loss for words.

IF YOU WANT	HERE'S WHAT YOU CAN SAY
...to probe for more information	• What are your ideas on that subject? • If you could choose, what would you like it to be? • Does anyone else have a thought about this? • Can you tell us a little more about that? • Jim brings up a good point. What do the rest of you think? • What is it about this issue that interests (or bothers) you? • Let's dream about what it would be like in a perfect world. • That idea has many dimensions. Can you tell us more about how it would work in our situation?
...to transition or segue to another topic	• Could you state that comment as a goal? • I'm glad you asked that question. Group, what do you think? • That comment has come up a lot. Should we explore it? • Are we in agreement? If so, let's move to the next issue. • Can someone summarize what we've accomplished here? • That's a great idea. Can anyone add to it? • Tell us why you find that idea so appealing (or useful).
...to stifle an interruption	• Let's put that in the *Parking Lot* so we can stay focused. That way, we'll remember to get back to it later. • How does this relate to the issue on the table? What's the link? • Let's check the minutes. I think we resolved that last week.
...to draw input from a quiet person or expert	• Sue, you know a lot about that; if you have any ideas, jump in. • Off the top of your head, does anybody feel differently? • I just want to hear anything that comes to your mind. • To an expert: How should I word this? What's your recommendation? How do you feel about that? • To a shy person: Keep talking. I want to hear more about this.
...to bring closure and summarize	• Can someone summarize what we've agreed to as a group? • Does anyone have anything else to add? • Are we in agreement? Let's go around the room and confirm. • We've got 5 minutes left. Let's brainstorm and multivote to list and prioritize the highlights of our discussion.

ADMINISTRATIVE STRUCTURE

Problem solving and the performance improvement process

The goal is to continuously improve performance results. The **Performance Improvement Action Path (PIAP)**, a.k.a. **CQI,** is the scientific process that leads to sustained improvements. It works best when there is total organizational commitment (i.e., every individual is responsible for quality and improving quality in his or her work) and a thoughtfully designed infrastructure.

1. **Administrative structure**—This document defines and describes the structure.
2. **Teamwork** —Teams help identify and remove obstacles.
3. **Technical Skills** —The PIAP (or any scientific or methodical problem solving process) and group process tools. Phases of the PIAP:
   - **Project Selection:** Identify and clarify improvement project.
   - **Cause Analysis & Evidence:** Seek root cause and verify with data.
   - **Solution Plan & Pilot:** Action plan and pilot improvement.
   - **Check, Adjust, Set Standard:** Confirm results, tweak, standardize, and implement.
4. **Factors most influential to the success of the PIAP (CQI) process**
   - Voluntary participation
   - Support of first-line supervisors
   - Top management support
   - Mid-management support/involvement

Quality Council

- Senior team (administration) preferred for first year of implementation
- Prevents systemic defects
- Demonstrates commitment
- Determines/communicates strategic direction (mission, vision, values, goals, strategies, rules)
- Enlists support from all organizational systems

Initial issues for the Quality Council

- What guidelines are needed to help the steering committee in their day-to-day functions?
- How many teams? Which departments? Cross-functional, natural, both? Who will be the facilitators? Team leaders? How will the process be communicated to all employees?
- What meeting space will be provided? What equipment (monitors, flipcharts) is needed? How will it be supplied? Where will the funds come from?
- What will training cover? What will be the schedule for training and initiating teams? When will teams meet, and what will compensation be?
- How will results be measured (participation, buy-in, problem resolution, financial gains)? Who will be accountable? How will recognition be handled?

Assessment & Strategic Implementation Planning for the Organization

- **Leadership & culture:** Vision, structure, readiness check, & accountability
- **Operations planning:** For implementation, rollout, maintaining the momentum
- **Financial planning:** Resource availability and affordability, budget, and return on investment
- **Education & training:** Needs analysis, scheduling, measurement of results
- **Communication:** Overall, ongoing, interdisciplinary
- **Systems integration & support:** Performance, measurement, planning, performance improvement, etc. How will systems be redesigned to support the performance improvement process?

(continues)

ADMINISTRATIVE STRUCTURE

(CONTINUED)

Charter - A written document detailing decisions made by the Quality Council

1. Philosophy & goals: Mission, vision, values, and goals of the QI process

    a. Mission   b. Vision   c. Values   d. Goals   e. Strategy

2. Program organization

    a. General principles   b. Support/steering committee

    c. Coordinator & facilitators   d. Teams and their operation

3. Teams and their operation

    a. Types of teams (Regular versus designated • Multi-issue versus single task • Different levels • Voluntary versus mandatory • Single versus mixed work units)

    b. Operation (size, membership, length of meetings, frequency, compensation, registration, leadership, skills, leaving a team…)

    c. Teams <u>can</u> work on these issues: Product quality, process improvement, reducing rework & operating costs, safety, scheduling, communication, morale…

    d. Teams <u>cannot</u> work on these issues: Grievances, seniority, pay, etc.

4. Responsibilities in problem solving or performance improvement (CQI)

    a. **Senior management**: Use it, plan for implementation, walk the talk, provide input, support, deploy problems and issues down the organization.

    b. **Mid-level management**: All of the above, plus

        • Get trained, learn about improvement teams, understand management's role.

        • Use group process tools (lead natural work team, be a member, use in committees).

        • Lead teams (help team work effectively, serve, and facilitate).

        • Interact with teams (support & influence, attend meetings occasionally, make presentations, maintain contact with team leader, read minutes).

        • Share implementation responsibility fairly, make realistic promises, follow through.

        • Supply recognition & reward on a timely, equitable basis (formal and informal).

        • Create supportive personnel policies.

        • Align and work with other departments/managers ("just the way we work here").

        • Miscellaneous things managers can do to help teams succeed: publicize and promote, get out of the way, offer ideas and advice, bridge to top management.

    c. **Employees**: Participate, use it, help peers, send problems to appropriate level/department.

    d. **Steering committee:** (See next page.)

    e. **Facilitators**: A pivotal role responsible for launching the process, training members and leaders, communicating, supporting, sustaining, monitoring, coaching, guiding.

        • Join steering committee.   • Take care of team training/organizational needs.

        • Recruit new teams.   • Serve as liaison to senior management.

        • Maintain team activity records.   • Prepare new training materials.

        • Arrange for program publicity.   • Help disband teams (outlived their usefulness).

        • Keep abreast of new ideas.   • See that day-to-day program needs are met.

    f. **Team leaders**: Responsible for the pacing and output of the team. Although employees are eligible to be team leaders, generally, they are managing the team.

(continues)

ADMINISTRATIVE STRUCTURE

Readiness factors – Indicators that the organization is ready to empower teams
- Both management and work force are receptive to participative management.
- Everyone is aware that with careful planning, unnecessary crises can be prevented.
- A department fits teamwork into existing work schedule, compensates, or shifts workload.
- All managers and supervisors have had at least a half-day orientation to the process.
- Active support from upper levels is in place.
- Facilitator support is provided.
- Ongoing training is accepted as the norm, and information is available to those who need it.
- Union support is possible.

Steering (or support) committee functions/responsibilities (10 to 12 members)

- Track events and accomplishments.
- Link levels, departments, functions.
- Facilitate implementation.
- Resolve defects in the system itself.
- Develop, deploy, and enforce policy guidelines.
- Review, support, and sustain the performance improvement process.

Steering committee composition (seek those with a systemwide perspective)

- Both sexes, major racial/ethnic groups, different age/seniority groups
- Different level of management and nonmanagement (including unions)
- A diversity of line departments and quality-related committees
- Strongly affected staff departments

Miscellaneous

- **Announce leader selection criteria in advance. If exception is selected, state why**
  - Enthusiastic about the process
  - Comfortable with people
  - Well organized
  - A volunteer
  - Interested in the development of others and able to support and encourage others
  - Knowledgeable about the techniques and willing to fill in the gaps over time

- **Code of conduct (examples of ground rules)**
  - Respect each person.
  - Criticize ideas, not people.
  - Ask questions and participate.
  - Listen with an open mind.
  - Share responsibilities.
  - Learn and practice skills & techniques.
  - Attend all sessions and be on time.
  - Strive to be an equal participant in the team.

- **Team member orientation**

  When a new team is chartered, offer training. Minimal orientation should include:
  - Greetings, introductions, and ground rules
  - Team work: Why is it important? What are problem solving/performance improvement teams and what is their purpose? How are they set up in your organization?
  - Performance Improvement Action Path Overview, including goals, key questions, specific steps, and responsibilities

FREQUENTLY ASKED QUESTIONS

- **Who should be members of the Quality Council (QC)?** Senior management (top administrators) and, when available (and appropriate), a Board representative and a medical staff officer.

- **What are the primary roles and responsibilities of the QC?** (1) Setting strategic direction for improving organizational performance; (2) creating policy, procedures, and operating guidelines (bylaws); and (3) guiding teams through the CQI process.

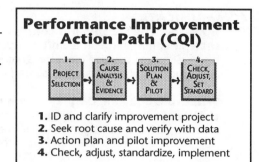

Performance Improvement Action Path (CQI)

1. PROJECT SELECTION → 2. CAUSE ANALYSIS & EVIDENCE → 3. SOLUTION PLAN & PILOT → 4. CHECK, ADJUST, SET STANDARD

1. ID and clarify improvement project
2. Seek root cause and verify with data
3. Action plan and pilot improvement
4. Check, adjust, standardize, implement

- **Should the QC establish a mission, vision, or goals for their team?** Although not required, every team can benefit from knowing their purpose and where they are headed. Also, identifying specific outcomes to achieve adds focus to the group's direction and provides an indicator for measuring results.

- **What are some of the initial priorities for the QC?**
(1) Prioritizing goals and agreeing on how the organization will approach improving organizational performance, (2) planning for a successful implementation, (3) ensuring that organizational systems are in place to support data management and measurement (for Joint Commission, assessing information system needs, PI support); efficient, consistent communication; and equity in the way rewards and recognitions are given.

- **What should the QC accomplish when its members meet? How involved should they be in the actual process? For example, to what extent should sponsors participate in the team process?** Their focus should be on strategic decision making and policy setting and helping teams progress. For the cross-functional teams, that will mean guidance and direction. For the natural work teams, it may mean only logging their process as an FYI. Sponsor participation is situational, depending on its potential positive contribution to the teamwork.

- **How often should the QC meet? Should there be a set agenda?** Initially, every 1 to 2 weeks (depending on the agenda requirements). Monthly meetings may be sufficient after 6 to 8 months, after strategies have been defined, and the focus is on tracking, guiding, and assisting teams. A set agenda may be difficult at first, due to the volume and variety of decisions that need to be addressed. However, the agenda should focus on two concerns: (1) decisions and policy and (2) cross-functional team progress. In time, as this becomes "the way you do business," meetings will settle into a routine format, and an agenda can be standardized.

- **What issues are appropriate for teams to pursue?** If subject matter experts are available, any issues related to improving care or service outcomes can be addressed, such as process improvements, reducing rework and operating costs, safety, scheduling, communication, and even morale. Issues like grievances, seniority, union issues, and salary are usually taboo.

- **What criteria can be used to prioritize issues?** See attached: Prioritizing Projects.

- **How many cross-functional teams can an organization support (afford) and how do we keep the rest of the organization motivated and involved?** For hospitals under 100 beds, 1 to 2 cross-functional teams will usually be the most that the organization can afford. Larger hospitals can manage 3 to 4 broad teams without creating a brain-drain on the organization. The rest of the organization is still involved in performance improvement activities via its natural work teams and its assigned work responsibilities.

(continues)

FREQUENTLY ASKED QUESTIONS

COMMUNICATION

- **How does the QC role get communicated to the members of the organization?** The strategic communication team/task force usually determines how this will be accomplished, however, many creative ideas have worked, from videotape to town meetings, to newsletters and brochures, to "open agenda" staff meetings with the administrator and quality coordinator.

- **What role does the QC play in communicating information about quality-related activities throughout the organization?** General information is shared as determined above, however, QC members, in their dual role as administrators, have other opportunities in day-to-day operations to communicate and reinforce information related to performance improvement.

- **How can the QC demonstrate and communicate its commitment to the process?** Walk the talk. Walk the talk. Walk the talk. Be a role model. Also, respond to those who are watching for evidence of change in senior management's behavior, actions, and decisions.

- **Who (which teams) are accountable to the QC?** It's situational; however, most organizations initially designate teams with three or more functions involved as a cross-functional team that must report in to the QC. The "reporting in" may be an FYI or a detailed progress report at the end of each phase of the QI process. Additionally, some organizations ask all teams, including natural work teams, to keep the QC abreast of their team activities so their projects can be logged and communicated to senior management and other departments. Typically, the Quality Coordinator is the point person who helps teams interact appropriately with the QC.

- **Where (to whom) does the team report results and progress?** Natural work teams report progress and results via their normal chain of command as they would any other work-related issue. Some organizations, however, initially ask natural work teams to report in (FYI) briefly on a standard format, so organizationwide progress can be captured and reported.

  Cross-functional teams are different in that they must report, formally, through the QC (sometimes via the QI coordinator) after each phase of the problem solving process (project selection, cause analysis and evidence, etc.). Each team member should also be keeping his or her natural work team manager abreast of team actions, to ensure maximum flow of information in and out of the team and coordination of all activities.

- **What method does the team use to keep the QC or senior management (administration) informed and current? What method is used to give feedback to the team?** It varies, but a common element is a standard written format. The team leader usually communicates with the quality coordinator or directly to the QC.

- **What content should be reported to the organization and to the Board?** (1) Progress report for the most recently completed phase and (2) measurable results.

TRAINING

- **What role does the QC play in defining continued CQI training to facilitate the housewide implementation plan? And what role do the facilitators play?** The QC determines the direction and strategic objectives for the organization's implementation of CQI and must then look to its management staff to assess if there are any unsatisfied educational needs. Thus, QC members must first set an expectation for the facilitator group and, second, hold the facilitators accountable for educating and coaching team leaders.

GENERAL

- **Who determines how quality-related participation will be assessed in performance evaluations? How?** Employees and managers should define their own outcome indicators, as well as the process (and indicators) they will follow to reliably and predictably achieve their desired outcomes. Measurable indicators also expedite evaluation and self-assessment.

PRIORITIZING PROJECTS

TYPE OF TEAM

Pilot
(a.k.a. jump start)

Three criteria are key for pilot teams: (1) Are we reasonably confident that this is an issue we can sink our teeth into and resolve? (2) Is there enough meat to the issue to convince others that the scientific method really works? (3) Is it a process that the leadership team can study, learn from, and use for implementation planning purposes?

Cross-functional

To some extent, every issue or process is cross-functional. However, some issues and processes involve several functions (or departments), and when something isn't working, the negative impact on outcomes and frustration can grow exponentially with each additional function. As natural work teams continue to crash into the *medical records process* or the *purchasing process* (for example) it becomes clear that these processes should be prioritized for immediate resolution so natural work teams can use them to help resolve their related issues.

Natural work
(a.k.a. home teams)

The scientific method or CQI is a proactive way to manage departments. Every department, or unit, is a natural work team, and the manager is the team leader. Successful managers probe their team ongoing: (1) <u>What</u> do we want to achieve to be most effective? (2) <u>How</u> will we get there? What is the best and most efficient process? (3) Can we afford that process within our <u>cost</u> <u>constraints</u>?

SELECTING THE RIGHT PROJECT

EVALUATION CRITERIA →

↓ POTENTIAL PROJECTS	Doable in 3 months?	Controllable by team?	Right members on team or available?	Team enthusiasm?	Measurable results?	Increases employee satisfaction?	Management support?	A successful solution will convert skeptics?	High probability of success?	Positive return on invest?	Timeliness factor?
ED patient waiting time			✓	✓			✓		✓	✓	
Admission/discharge process	✓	✓	✓	✓	✓		✓	✓	✓	✓	✓
Patient flow							✓		✓	✓	
Lost patient articles	✓			✓		✓		✓	✓		
MIA medical records			✓				✓				
Employee evaluation process			✓	✓	✓	✓		✓			
Reporting/analyzing injuries	✓					✓		✓	✓		
Infection prevention process	✓	✓		✓		✓			✓		
Medication delivery process		✓	✓	✓	✓	✓	✓	✓	✓	✓	
Purchasing process					✓	✓		✓	✓		

TEAM START-UP & TRACKING FORM

Date _____

Project title _____

Project goal/vision _____
_____

Improvement payoff potential:

❑ *Customer satisfaction (check one):* ❑ *Patient* ❑ *Employee* ❑ *Physician* ❑ *External*

❑ *Cost containment or productivity gain*

❑ *Process streamlining and simplification*

❑ *Other (explain)* _____

Chartered by _____ **Sponsor** _____

Start date _____ **Expected completion date** _____

Meeting day/time _____ **Meeting length** _____

Facilitator _____ **Team leader** _____

Team members _____ _____

_____ _____

_____ _____

_____ _____

_____ _____

Type of team *(check all that apply)*

❑ *Assigned/mandated* ❑ *Voluntary* ❑ *Natural work team* ❑ *Cross-functional*

Prescheduled routine check-ins

Who _____ When *(list dates)* _____

Phases of problem solving or process improvement *(fill in completion dates)*

- *Project selection*   Target date _____   Actual _____
- *Cause analysis & evidence* Target date _____   Actual _____
- *Solution planning & pilot* Target date _____   Actual _____
- *Check, adjust, standardize* Target date _____   Actual _____

Please attach outcome indicators and measurement results as they become available.

TEAM START-UP & TRACKING FORM

When pursuing a scientific approach to problem solving or process improvement, each phase of the process must be completed before work begins on the next phase (i.e., no solution seeking until the root cause is verified). Briefly, document completion of each phase. Attach data or tools as needed.

Project Selection *phase output: (1) Write a concise statement of the project below. (2) Attach a breakdown of the "avoidable cost of quality," i.e., what it costs the organization, in dollars, when quality targets aren't met... and we have to pay the price.*

_____

_____

_____

_____

_____

Cause Analysis and Evidence *phase output: Describe the root cause of the problem or the breakdown in the process. Attach data to support your assumption(s).*

_____

_____

_____

_____

_____

Solution Planning and Pilot *phase output: List three solutions that have the best potential for (1) resolving the problem/breakdown and (2) a successful implementation. Attach a cost-benefit analysis (for each) and an action plan for implementing the selected solution.*

_____

_____

_____

_____

_____

Check, Adjust, Standardize *phase output: List three indicators that will be measured and monitored ongoing. These indicators must be able to verify whether or not the implemented solution, or new process, is working and outcomes are being met.*

_____

_____

_____

_____

_____

TEAM START-UP & TRACKING FORM

Joint Commission's Dimensions of Performance

To the sponsoring person/group: Guide the team in a worthwhile direction by setting clear parameters. Mark the quality indicators to be addressed in the improvement project. Other parameters might include: target cost; amount of time and target dates for check-in, feedback, and completion; composition of team, (i.e., which departments, who, how many); required data; available resources; and expectations in general.

Doing the Right Thing

❏ The **efficacy** of the procedure or treatment in relation to the patient's condition – The degree to which the care/intervention for the patient has been shown to accomplish the desired/projected outcome(s)

❏ The **appropriateness** of a specific test, procedure, or service to meet the patient's needs – The degree to which the care/intervention provided is relevant to the patient's clinical needs, given the current state of knowledge

Doing the Right Thing Well

❏ The **availability** and **accessibility** of a needed test, procedure, treatment, or service to the patient who needs it – The degree to which appropriate care/intervention is available to meet the patient's needs

❏ The **timeliness** with which a needed test, procedure, treatment, or service is provided to the patient – The degree to which the care/intervention is provided to the patient at the most beneficial or necessary time

❏ The **effectiveness** with which tests, procedures, treatments, and services are provided – The degree to which the care/intervention is provided in the correct manner, given the current state of knowledge, in order to achieve the desired/projected outcome for the patient

❏ The **continuity** of the services provided to the patient with respect to other services, practitioners, and providers, and over time – The degree to which the care/intervention for the patient is coordinated among practitioners, among organizations, and over time

❏ The **safety** of the patient (and others) to whom the services are provided – The degree to which the risk of an intervention and the risk in the care environment are reduced for the patient and others, including the healthcare provider

❏ The **efficiency** with which services are provided – The relationship between the outcomes (results of care) and the resources used to deliver patient care

❏ The **respect and caring** with which services are provided – The degree to which the patient or a designee is involved in his/her own care decisions and to which those providing services to do so with sensitivity and respect for the patient's needs, expectations, and individual differences

❏
_____

❏
_____

SOURCE: Joint Commission. **1996 Accreditation Manual for Hospitals: Volume I • Standards** Oakbrook Terrace, IL: JCAHO, 1996. p. 102. Used with permission.

STAGES OF TEAM GROWTH[9, 10]

Forming Excitement, optimism, pride, some fear—define task and how to achieve it

Storming Resistance, conflict, attitude fluctuations—competition choosing sides, unrealistic goals, questioning wisdom of those who selected the issue and other members

Norming Harmony, cohesion, team spirit, and group norms—expressing constructive criticism, focus on goals and outcome

Performing Constructive self-change, solving/preventing problems, systems thinking, tight team, achieving breakthrough

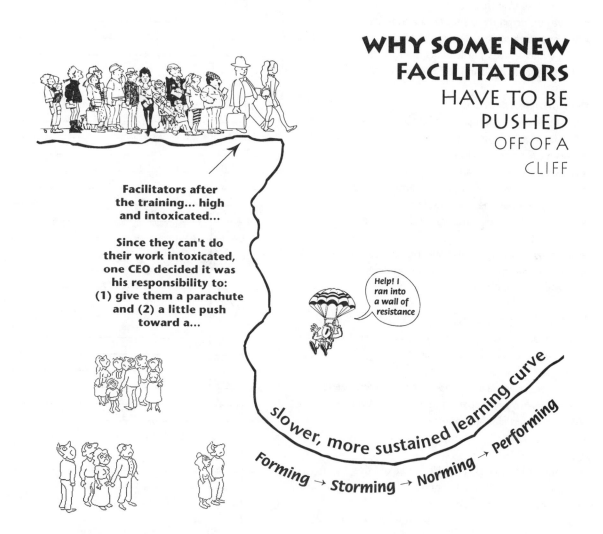

WHY SOME NEW FACILITATORS
HAVE TO BE PUSHED
OFF OF A CLIFF

Facilitators after the training... high and intoxicated...

Since they can't do their work intoxicated, one CEO decided it was his responsibility to: (1) give them a parachute and (2) a little push toward a...

Help! I ran into a wall of resistance

slower, more sustained learning curve

Forming → Storming → Norming → Performing

ᴀCILITATOR SKILLS CHECKLIST

r* Competencies	Not Met	Met	Exceeded	Improvement Ideas

ˌs Skills
- ᴏup issues and concerns
- ᴜ. , positive opening (with relevant background info)
- Establɪ. ɪes a clear, but flexible agenda related to group issues
- Structures and guides the session to reach objectives
- Shows flexibility in adapting materials or methods
- Creates an atmosphere of openness and trust
- Attends to the group's emotional undercurrents
- Acknowledges and reinforces group participation
- Helps group members confront each other, as needed, and reach consensus
- Moves participants to specific action steps
- Serves as a catalyst for the application of concepts and skills
- Paces and moves participants along with smooth transitions that clarify, bring to closure, link to next topic

Presentation Skills
- Shows energy, enthusiasm, and empathy
- Demonstrates mastery of process
- Uses a supportive and motivating style
- Appears natural and sincere
- Uses humor well and supports learning objectives
- Varies voice volume, tone, and pace appropriately
- Uses effective body language and movement
- Speaks clearly and to the point
- Supports learning points with concrete examples
- Creates clear, visually stimulating flipcharts
- Uses audiovisual aids effectively

Communication Skills
- Asks effective questions (open- and close-ended)
- Actively listens and responds accordingly
- Uses self-disclosure appropriately
- Confronts people in a supportive way when needed
- Receives group feedback and uses it positively
- Engages participants appropriately off-line

Personal Skills
- Establishes personal credibility and expertise
- Appears genuinely confident, with humility and modesty
- Develops rapport and earns trust
- Shows respect and interest toward participants
- Coordinates session logistics
- Follows through on commitments and agreements

*These competencies are also applicable to team leaders and quality coordinators.

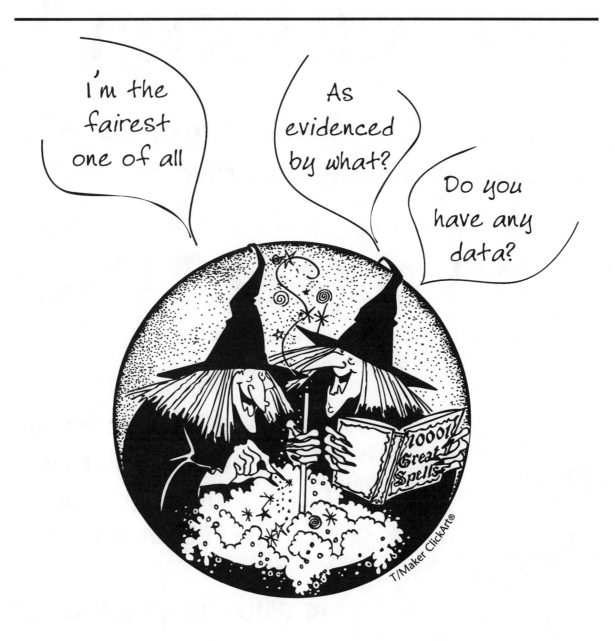

Indicators provide evidence...
of **where** you're going, **how** to get there,
and **how well** you're doing

Are You Lonely?

If you hate the responsibility of working alone and making your own decisions

Call a MEETING

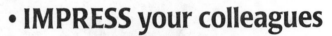

YOU CAN...
- IMPRESS your colleagues
- DRAW on flipcharts
- MEET people
- FEEL important

BE PAID FOR HANGING OUT

MEETINGS

The relaxing alternative to work

Revised from an unknown source

TYPES OF TEAMS

	Cross-Functional	Task Force	Department Level
Goal	Improve a process across three or more departments.	Complete a one-time self-contained activity or task.	Continuously improve department operations.
Membership Who	Usually voluntary - A cross-section of process owners: employees, physicians, customers	Usually voluntary - A cross-section of process owners: employees, physicians, customers	Mandatory - Department employees and others as needed and appropriate
Size	6–8 members	6–8 members	8–12 members
Project selected by and team accountable to	Quality Council prioritized by customer feedback	Quality Council prioritized by customer feedback	Department manager and employees
Life Cycle	10–20 meetings	5–10 meetings	Ongoing
Meeting length	2–4 hours (and longer, as needed)	1–2 hours	1–1.5 hours on rotating shifts
Data collection responsibility	Team members and designated resources	Team members and designated resources	Team members and designated resources
Solution implementation responsibility	Senior managers Physicians Dept. managers	Senior managers Physicians Dept. managers	Dept. managers Team members
Recommended leader	Experienced facilitator	Facilitator or team leader	Dept. manager or his or her designee

TEAMS

What works

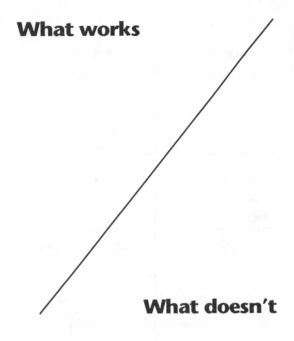

What doesn't

Management's role

- ■ *Learn* and *use* tools & concepts.
- ■ *Lead* and *interact* with teams, other functions/depts., managers.
- ■ Identify team leader & **structure.**
- ■ Select team members or **criteria.**
- ■ Identify **goal, process,** resources.
- ■ Create supportive **policies.**
- ■ Share **implementation** responsibility.
- ■ *Empower, recognize, reward.*

Roles & responsibilities

Team Leaders:

- ■ Keep discussion moving **forward.**
- ■ Bring group back from **tangents.**
- ■ Question to **open/close discussion.**
- ■ Encourage **equal input.**
- ■ Help group reach **consensus.**

Facilitators:

- ■ All of the above, **plus...**
- ■ **Educate/train** team leaders.
- ■ **Assess** team leader **skills.**
- ■ Coach leaders on **improvements.**
- ■ **Communicate** with Quality Council.

Team leader selection criteria

- ■ Rated highly on **appraisals**
- ■ Knows organization, **how it works**
- ■ Interested and **motivated**
- ■ **Brings out the best** in others
- ■ Earned **credibility** and respect
- ■ Demonstrated **commitment**
- ■ Optimistic, positive about **value**
- ■ Energetic and **self-confident**
- ■ Awareness of **group process**
- ■ Use of the **scientific** approach

TEAM SUCCESS

10 Ingredients for a successful team[11]

- *Clarity in team **goals***
- *An improvement **plan***
- *Clearly defined **roles***
- *Clear **communication***
- *Beneficial team **behaviors***
- *Well-defined decision **procedures***
- *Balanced **participation***
- *Established **ground rules***
- *Awareness of **group process***
- *Use of the **scientific** approach*

When to pass on a team

- *Support from **senior management** or the **process owners** is lacking.*
- *Return on investment information cannot **demonstrate the need**.*
- ***Culture** is not conducive.*
- ***Information** is unavailable.*
- ***Team leader skills** are lacking.*
- *Members are **unprepared** or **decline**.*
- ***Reward system** is inadequate.*
- *Focus conflicts with current **strategy***

How senior management can help

- *Clear, well-communicated **goals***
- *Real and visible **involvement***
- *Adequate **time** for the task*
- *Pertinent **feedback***
- *Adequate **training**/preparation*
- *Cooperative **behavior** model*
- *Focused, nonjudgmental **attention***
- *Even, shared **participation***
- *Flinch-free **empowerment***
- *Routine use of **group process***
- *Clearly defined **parameters***

Setting clear parameters: Some examples

- ***Expectations** in general*
- ***Target cost** or cost-benefit ratio*
- ***Time** to be spent by the team*
- *Number of **team members** and often **who** will be members*
- ***Departments** or **people** to be **included** or interviewed*
- ***Data** to review and analyze*
- ***Resources** available to the team (training, labor, supplies, etc.)*
- *Target points to **check-in** and provide **feedback** to authority*

MAKING THE MOST OF MEETINGS

Facilitators are responsible for helping team leaders learn how to manage and make the most of (very expensive) meeting time. If you don't have time to read all the books on managing meetings, this information may be helpful.

Focus	Process
Up-front agreements	• Have the group create and adhere to ground rules. For example, set an expectation that meetings will begin and end on time. Then do it! And don't repeat or summarize discussion for latecomers. • Make sure team members want to be there and that their supervisors actively support their participation. • Have team members sign off on their responsibility statements. • Review expectations of team output, including their primary objective and target date for completion.
Planning and preparation	• Use square or round tables to create an "equal" environment. • Use "U" shape for teaching. • Have 2-3 flipcharts (and markers) on hand, ready for use. • Create an action-focused agenda with time allocations noted. • Brief invited guests on the meeting format and expectations. • Preprint any announcements and attach to the agenda. • Cancel the meeting if it's not necessary and if nothing is to be gained from meeting.
During the meeting	• Use group process tools to equalize participation and efficiently move the group's work forward. • Allocate 5 minutes for an ice breaker, and put it first on the agenda. • Ask for a volunteer to be the keeper of the ground rules. He or she will spend most of his or her time bringing people back from tangents. • Actively listen and acknowledge input. • Ask open questions to bring out discussion and closed questions to focus the group, bring them to consensus, or move them forward. • Use the flipchart to process and document key information. It will be enormously helpful in pulling together the minutes. • Give verbal and nonverbal cues on how time is progressing.
Follow up	• Always do what you say you're going to do. • Document results and outside assignments. Check in with team members between assignments to see if they need help. • Involve team members in setting and addressing the agenda. • Briefly critique meeting as a group or by a short survey form. • Ask for volunteers to debrief with and solicit input from stakeholders who are not team members prior to the next meeting.

AGENDA CHECKLIST

Many team leaders consider the agenda as their strategic meeting plan <u>and</u> key to success. Think of the last few meetings for which you were responsible (team meeting, staff meeting, Cub Scout meeting) and check (R) the actions you routinely include on your agendas. Then identify (√) the actions you haven't tried, but want to add to your routine for your next meeting agenda.

WHO _____ ■ *Name of the group*
_____ ■ *Person calling or responsible for the meeting*
_____ ■ *Guest, observer, or guest resource person*
_____ ■ *Person responsible for agenda changes*

WHY _____ ■ *Routine or special meeting*
_____ ■ *Background information (if needed)*

WHAT _____ ■ *Agenda sent prior to meeting (2–10 days)*
_____ ❑ *Meeting purpose, goal, or desired outcomes*
_____ ❑ *Action items listed in order of priority*
_____ ❑ *Person responsible for the action item noted*
_____ ❑ *Process to be used on action item (report, brainstorming, data display, presentation, discussion)*
_____ ❑ *Time allocated for each action item*

WHERE _____ ■ *Location (including room number if needed)*

WHEN _____ ■ *Day, date, time (include both start & end times)*

OTHER _____ ■ *Decision parameters or limits known by group*
_____ ■ *Ground rules established and posted*
_____ ■ *Preparation: Prereading, background materials, or other things to bring to meeting*

SAMPLE GROUND RULES

Ground rules are simply a list of behavior guidelines, created by the team at their first meeting as they agree on how they will work together. They are posted at every meeting. Some of the most popular ground rules are listed below, but every team has a different list. The process of creating the ground rules is as important as the finished product, so take the necessary time to create your own.

❑ **Attendance**
  - When meetings will be held (agree on a regular day and time).
  - Where meetings will be held (seek a regular space and schedule ahead).
  - Attendance is required unless excused by the team leader.
  - Three unexcused absences will end the tenure of the team member.
  - All meetings will begin and end on time.

❑ **Pacing and time management**
  - Agendas will be set in time frames, and every effort will be made to work within the chosen time allocation.
  - A timekeeper will be assigned (a rotating position) to provide time information and keep team members "on track."

❑ **Participation and communication**
  - Equal participation is expected for both meetings and assignments.
  - Responsibility and resources will be shared on assignments.
  - Assignments will be ready on time, and members will be adequately prepared for meetings, so that meetings can be productive.
  - Routine chores or duties (recorder, meeting arranger, etc.) will be rotated.
  - Candid open discussions will be encouraged... and held as confidential.
  - One person speaks at a time without interruption.
  - Stay open to new ideas. No judging or criticizing ideas.
  - Clarify what's okay to talk about and what's not.

❑ **Documentation**
  - Agendas for the next meeting will be created at the end of every meeting.
  - Time will be allocated for each action step by the team.
  - Minutes will document the team's activities. Members will rotate this role.
  - The facilitator or team leader will be responsible for distributing minutes.

❑ **Group behavior**
  - It's okay to disagree. Conflicts will be open and resolved by the team.
  - Once consensus is reached, all will support the team decision.

❑ **Miscellaneous**
  - Beepers, phones, and other retrieval devices will be checked at the door.
  - If a meeting is longer than 2 hours, there will be a break and refreshments.
  - Access to resources, support services, equipment, and supplies will be coordinated through the team leader or the facilitator.
  - The team leader is responsible for room setup.
  - Everyone is responsible for cleanup.

Action Meeting Minutes

Conclusions: The team reached consensus on two possible root causes of outpatient delays: (1) the prescheduling and preregistration processes and (2) the high percentage of "walk-in" patients. The decision was made to collect supporting data to drive future decisions.

Recommendations: Create (1) a data collection form for monitoring outpatient waiting times and (2) a log for tracking the workload of registration clerks. All data will be analyzed and evaluated by the whole team for future use.

Objective What are the expected results?	Action How will results be accomplished? Specifically, what steps will be taken? How will results be measured?	Resources Labor, supply, and equipment costs	• Completion Date (When) • Responsible Person (Who)
A data collection form for monitoring outpatient waiting times *Agenda: 25 minutes*	• List all actions related to scheduling, preregistering, and completing procedures. • Create a written survey and try it. • Teach registration clerks how to use the form that will document patient waiting times and help identify the bottleneck. **Indicator:** Areas of waiting time exceeding an acceptable range will be identified and then analyzed for resolution.	• 3 hours meeting time for 3-4 team members for survey development • 1 hour for training 4 registration clerks	• **When:** 7/1/92 • **Who:** Outpatient dept. managers, registration clerks, and team members Jeff & Jessica
Written log of registration clerk workload *Agenda: 20 minutes*	• Registration clerks will log workload activities and the actual time required to accomplish tasks (time period: 2 weeks). • Team will analyze data and take action. **Indicator:** Prioritized list of registration tasks and required hours of workload	• Activity logs • 20 minutes documentation time daily	• **When:** 7/15/92 • **Who:** Registration clerks
Written update of team activity for: **- Mgmt. Council or** **- Quality Council** *Agenda: 10 minutes*	• Team members log targeted results and action steps in meeting minutes. • Communicate progress to management council and the hospitalwide quality assessment and improvement team. **Indicator:** An update will be given on team activities each Friday in the bulletin	• Team meeting minutes • Hours to produce/distribute written report • Team member representation at meetings	• **When:** Weekly • **Who:** Team members, news staff, and print shop personnel
Progress report sent and feedback received from peers and management after each team meeting *Homework: 30 minutes*	• Post meeting minutes on unit bulletin board. • Gather specific feedback for the next team meeting: acceptance, recommended revisions, suggestions for "next steps." - Review at monthly unit staff meeting - Meet with unit manager individually **Indicator:** Employees actively participate in CQI process by listing recommendations or initialing acceptance of proposed changes.	• 1 hour for staff meeting • 1 hour for meeting with manager	• **When:** Next team meeting (ongoing) • **Who:** All team members

ASSESSING TEAM EFFECTIVENESS

Instructions: Rate your team on each of the following nine dimensions using a scale of 1 to 5, indicating your assessment of your team and the way it functions by circling the number on each scale that you feel is most descriptive of your team. Use every other month or when a problem arises.

1. Vision and Goals

1   2   3   4   5

Vision and goals are either not established, unclear, or unstable.

The team members understand, have agreed to, and support the team's vision and goals.

2. Resource Utilization (labor, supplies, equipment)

1   2   3   4   5

Team members are not acknowledged and/or utilized equally.

The resources of all team members are fully acknowledged, appreciated, and utilized.

3. Trust and Conflict Resolution

1   2   3   4   5

There is little trust among team members and conflict is ongoing.

There is a high degree of trust among team members and conflict is dealt with openly and resolved.

4. Leadership

1   2   3   4   5

Leadership is autocratic, undependable, and does not treat members equally.

Leadership uses team goals to guide and facilitate, dependably, and equally.

5. Meeting Process and Procedures

1   2   3   4   5

There is little control. Ground rules are not available and/or not followed.

There are effective ground rules created and supported by members and used to self-regulate.

6. 2-Way Communication (talking and listening)

1   2   3   4   5

Team members spout opinions and do not speak openly and honestly.

Team members reference facts and feel comfortable speaking openly and honestly.

7. Problem Solving and Decision Making

1   2   3   4   5

The team has does not use a standard process for problem solving/decision making.

The team follows a standard, data-driven approach to problem solving/decision making.

8. Risk Taking, Flexibility, Change

1   2   3   4   5

The team is inflexible and avoids looking at other alternatives, risky decisions, and changes.

The team is flexible, takes risks with different approaches, and seeks change and innovation.

9. Performance Assessment and Improvement

1   2   3   4   5

The team never evaluates its outcomes or process and never adjusts to improve.

The team evaluates its outcomes and processes frequently and makes adjustments to improve.

TEAM OBSERVER'S GUIDE

Instructions: Reflect on and score the team experience. This guide can be used at the end of meetings for feedback to the leader.

	No	Some	Yes
1) Did the **leadership** help the group stay on track?	①	②	③
2) Did everyone **participate**?	①	②	③
3) Were people **open** and sharing info?	①	②	③
4) Were ideas **responded** to with acceptance, interest, and without evaluation?	①	②	③
5) Was **consensus** used successfully (resulting in the group supporting the decision)?	①	②	③
6) **Two-way communication**: Were people actively listening—to tone of voice, body language, eye contact, questions, paraphrasing—as well as talking?	①	②	③
7) Were people direct? **Respectful**? **Assertive**?	①	②	③

TOTAL SCORE _____

FOR OBSERVERS AND DEBRIEFING:

WHAT CONTRIBUTED TO THE TEAM'S SUCCESS? PREVENTED SUCCESS? WHAT COULD HAVE GENERATED GREATER EFFECTIVENESS?

REWARD & RECOGNIZE

FREEBIES... OR VERY CLOSE
Managers are free to administer as desired

REWARDS UNDER $50
Managers can award with approval of direct supervisor

REWARDS OVER $50
Criteria based – administrative or committee approval required

IS THE BRAINSTORMED REWARD A FREEBIE, OVER $50, OR UNDER $50?

1.
2.
3.
4.
5.
6.
7.
8.
9.
10.
11.
12.
13.
14.
15.

1.
2.
3.
4.
14.
15.

This is a brainstorming activity to do with a group and a lot of flipchart paper. It can be facilitated two different ways:

1. Team leader writes all brainstormed ideas on a flipchart one at a time. Then, after the brainstorming, team members multivote to prioritize their favorites in each category by putting red "stick-on" dots on >$50, blue on <$50, and green on Freebies.

2. Team leader uses masking tape to place flipchart paper (2 layers to prevent wall damage) around the meeting room. One wall will be the Freebie Wall, another the <$50 wall, and the third the >$50 wall. During the meeting—or over a number of days—team members walk around the room and write their ideas on the appropriate wall. When the flipcharts are full of ideas, clarify, remove duplications, and let the group campaign for their favorites. Team members then multivote (5 multivotes per category) to prioritize and identify the best options in each category. This is called Wallstorming.

SPECIFICALLY, WHEN SHOULD WE USE FREEBIES, UNDER $50, AND OVER $50 TO PRAISE EFFORTS?

RECOGNITION IDEAS

Top picks:

Promotion and/or raise
When someone above me values
    my opinion
Special assignment
Time off/compensatory time
$50, or other monetary award
Verbal recognition (public or private)
Taken to lunch
Dinner at the boss' house
Employee of the quarter/year
Thank you (especially hand-written)
Family get-together
Attendance at a special training
Trading places with someone (at work)
    for a day

Other ideas:

Recognition and commendation by peers
Day off • Bonus pay
Exposure to upper management
Periodic review of job performance
Opportunities for continued education
Gift book inscribed by the top managers
Written recognition
Little button or stick-on: good job
Getting caught doing something right
Reward of more training/seminar
Memo to my boss' boss
Article in organization's newsletter
    or local newspaper story
Corporate mug, tie tack, etc.
Written summary of the value I bring
Atta boy/girl
Peer review and recognition
Gift/present
Ability to pick where I work
Higher management exposure
Invitation to become a facilitator
Manager giving credit to employee
Gift certificate (grocery, massage, nails,
    gym, come in late/leave early)
Gifts from local merchants

Add your ideas:

_____

_____

_____

_____

_____

_____

_____

_____

_____

_____

_____

_____

_____

_____

_____

_____

_____

_____

_____

CULTURE ASSESSMENT

Directions: This assessment has <u>two</u> <u>parts</u>. Using the scale to the right of the stated expectation, (1) rate your organization's performance by writing an "**A**" to indicate the **actual** performance. (2) On the same scale, write a "**U**" to indicate the **urgency** of the needed change; "5" is most urgent.

1. **Mission** – The overall purpose and philosophy of the organization and the extent to which staff members understand it, recognize its value to their work, and reference it to help make daily work decisions.

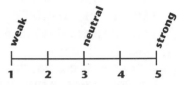

2. **Vision** – The extent to which leadership prepares for and shares the desired future of the organization and expected contributions of staff members.

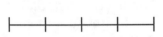

3. **Leadership** – The ability of management to coordinate, motivate, and engage staff members to achieve their goals and the vision of the organization.

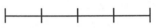

4. **Image** – How the organization is perceived by customers, employees, and the community. A strong image is favorably regarded by its community.

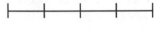

5. **Institutional pride** – The positive feelings and enthusiasm employees have for their work and their organization as a place to work or receive services.

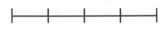

6. **Customer focus** – The extent to which individuals demonstrate personal responsibility in seeking out and responding to customer (patients, visitors, employees, physicians) needs and concerns.

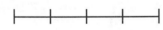

7. **Trust** – The extent to which people in the organization can count on each other as they pursue a common goal.

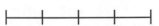

8. **Communication** – The clarity, openness, and timeliness of conveying information and plans throughout the organization.

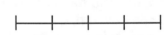

9. **Innovation and creativity** – The extent to which the organization initiates, responds to, and supports development of new ideas, different directions, and risk taking.

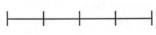

10. **Teamwork** – The cooperative effort of employees working within their work unit, or cross-functionally, to solve problems and prevent their recurrence in the future.

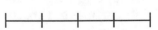

(continues)

CULTURE ASSESSMENT

(CONTINUED)

11. **Employee appreciation** – The extent to which the organization values its employees and their contribution to the service.

weak — neutral — strong
1   2   3   4   5

12. **Performance improvement** – The degree of commitment to excellence, the pursuit of doing the right things, the right way, the first time, throughout the organization.

13. **Rewards and recognition** – The extent to which staff members are equitably recognized for performance results, gains, and contributions.

14. **Responsibility and accountability** – The extent to which employee expectations are clearly stated and reviewed regularly by management.

15. **Employee involvement and participation** – The opportunity for employees to determine, or influence, how work processes they use will be performed.

16. **Capacity for change** – The ability of the organization to plan for, communicate, and manage ongoing change.

17. **"We have a quality company"** – Check your choice to indicate how you feel about the following statement:

    1. Strongly disagree
    2. Moderately disagree
    3. Agree
    4. Moderately agree
    5. Strongly agree

1   2   3   4   5

18. **Who are you?**

_____ Executive staff   _____ Management staff   _____ Educator
_____ Supervisory staff   _____ Staff member/employee

19. **Comments:**

Thank you for participating and completing this form.

NOTES

1. D. Wallechinsky et al., *The Book of Lists* (New York: William Morrow & Co., Inc., 1977).

2. J. W. Newstrom and E. Scannell, *Games Trainers Play* (New York: McGraw-Hill, 1980).

3. Newstrom and Scannell, *Games*.

4. Newstrom and Scannell, *Games*.

5. *Hospitals & Health Networks* (October 20, 1993): 37.

6. B.C. James, "Implementing Practice Guidelines Through Clinical Quality Improvement," *Frontiers of Health Services Management* (Fall 1993): 3–37.

7. A.B. Campbell and N.S. Lakier, *Healthcare Forum Journal* (July/August 1993): 81–83.

8. D.M. Berwick, "The Clinical Process and the Quality Process," *Quality Management in Health Care* (Fall 1992): 1–8.

9. B. Tuckman, "Development Sequence in Small Groups," *Psychological Bulletin* (1965): 284–399.

10. P. Scholtes, *The Team Handbook* (Madison, WI: Joiner Associates, Inc., 1988).

11. Scholtes, *Team Handbook*.

RECOMMENDED READING

Byham, W., with J. Cox. 1988 *Zapp! The lightning of empowerment.* New York: Harmony Books.

Denton, D.K. October 1992. Building a team. *Quality Progress.* 87–91.

🐦 Doyle, M., and D. Straus. 1976. *How to make meetings work: The new interaction method.* New York: Jove Books.

🐦 Harper, A., and B. Harper. 1992. *Skill-building for self-directed team members.* New York: MW Corporation.

Hiam, A. 1990. *The vest-pocket CEO: Decision-making tools for executives.* Englewood Cliffs, NJ: Prentice Hall.

Kohn, A. 1986. *No contest: The case against competition.* Boston: Houghton-Mifflin Company.

Lee, C. June 1990. Beyond teamwork. *Training.* 25–32.

Mill, C.R. 1989. *Activities for trainers: 50 Useful designs.* San Diego: University Associates.

Newstrom, J.W., and E. Scannell. 1980. *Games trainers play.* New York: McGraw-Hill.

Newstrom, J.W., and E. Scannell. 1983. *More games trainers play.* New York: McGraw-Hill.

Pfeiffer, W. 1989. *Encyclopedia of group activities: 150 Practical designs for successful facilitating.* San Diego: University Associates.

Rapaport, R. January–February 1993. To build a winning team: An interview with head coach Bill Walsh. *Harvard Business Review.* 111–120.

Sashkin, M. 1989. *Structured activities: Management training in communication.* King of Prussia, PA: Organization Design & Development, Inc.

Sisco, R. February 1993. What to teach team leaders. *Training.* 62–67.

🐦 Scholtes, P. 1988. *The team handbook: How to use teams to improve quality.* Madison, WI: Joiner Associates, Inc.

Wellins, R. et al. 1991. *Empowered teams.* San Francisco: Jossey-Bass.

🐦 *If you don't have time to read them all, read these first.*